School Nurse's

SURVIVAL GUIDE

Ready-to-Use Tips, Techniques
& Materials for the School
Health Professional

Richard M. Adams, M.D.
Director of Health Services, Dallas Public Schools

PRENTICE HALL
Paramus, New Jersey 07652

Library of Congress Cataloging-in-Publication Data

Adams, Richard M. (Richard Martin)
    School nurse's survival guide : ready-to-use tips, techniques, and
materials for the school health professional / by Richard M. Adams.
        p.   cm.
    Includes bibliographical references.
    ISBN 0-13-186727-X
    1. School nursing—Handbooks, manuals, etc.   I. Title.
RJ247.A33   1995   95-18454
371.7'12—dc20   CIP

Printed in the United States of America

10   9   8   7   6   5   4

ISBN 0-13-186727-X

ATTENTION: CORPORATIONS AND SCHOOLS

Prentice Hall books are available at quantity discounts with bulk purchase for
educational, business, or sales promotional use. For information, please write to:
Prentice Hall Career & Personal Development Special Sales, 240 Frisch Court,
Paramus, New Jersey 07652. Please supply: title of book, ISBN number,
quantity, how the book will be used, date needed.

PRENTICE HALL

Paramus, NJ 07652

On the World Wide Web at http://www.phdirect.com

DEDICATION

To the indomitable, unsinkable, gentle but unswerving
character of school nurses everywhere
and to
John D. Nelson, M.D., my first medical writing mentor. He helped me
gain my first journal byline by wielding a red pencil more terrible than
that of any English teacher. His modeling of brevity and clarity in
writing has stood me in good stead through the years.

ACKNOWLEDGMENTS

A number of people contributed significantly to this book by suggesting topics, critiquing chapters, translating forms into Spanish, typing manuscript pages, or simply providing moral support.

The major contributors I wish to thank (in no particular order) are: Marilyn Marcontel, Van Chauvin, Roscoe Lewis, Robert Haley, Phil Francis, JoAnne Duncan, Phyllis Simpson, Robert Mendro, Bertha Whatley, Dennis Eichelbaum, Eduardo Vargas, Alicia Rodriguez, Annie Orphey, Darlene English, Elaine Sheets, Cynthia Hanna, Elizabeth Jackson, Altonette Ford, Diana Aldape Walker, Caryl White, Sharon Reeves, Olivia Hernandez, Viola Gray, Jo Ellen Bogert, Deborah Chapel, Chad Woolery, Milton A. Cardwell, Jr., and Robert L. Johnston. Without the help of these individuals, you would not be holding this volume.

ABOUT THE AUTHOR

Richard M. Adams, M.D., (B.S. and M.D. degrees, Louisiana State University) serves as Director of Health Services for the Dallas Public Schools and for the past ten years has been a consultant to the High School for Health Professions. He is also Clinical Associate Professor of Pediatrics at Southwestern Medical School in Dallas and Clinical Associate Professor of Community Medicine at the University of Texas Health Science Center. He served two years as a major and Chief of Pediatrics at the Luke Air Force Base in Phoenix, Arizona.

Dr. Adams is a Diplomate of the American Board of Pediatrics, a member of the American School Health Association (former Vice Chairman of the Physician's Committee, and Assistant Editor for Medicine—*Journal of School Health*), the American Medical Writers Association and other organizations. He also serves on a number of boards and committees of health agencies, including Vice-Chairman, Advisory Committee on the Comprehensive School Health Program—Texas State Board of Education. He is past chairman of the Texas Council of Urban School Districts' Health Advisory Committee.

The author of numerous articles published in professional journals and textbooks, Dr. Adams lectures on school health at state and national conventions. He was honored in a ceremony at the White House for his immunization efforts in Dallas (May 1992).

FOREWORD

School nursing practice in the 90's is both broad and varied in scope. Today, the school nurse provides direct student health services; conducts health/wellness programs for school personnel; is involved in program planning, development, management and evaluation and provides health education and counseling for students as well as families. This highlights but some of the current challenges facing the nurse in the school setting.

With these varied role responsibilities it becomes easy to understand that in addition to clinical expertise the school nurse needs information on a wide variety of topics (i.e., financial, legal, environmental, etc.) as well as skill in research, political advocacy and public relations. The *School Nurse's Survival Guide* was written to provide the school nurse with a quick reference for practical and technical information on many such topics. While noting which areas are important to school nursing practice, the reader will be motivated to explore each topic in greater depth and detail.

I believe *School Nurse's Survival Guide* will be a practical resource manual for dealing with the challenges of providing health care in schools today.

Carole Passarelli RN, MS, CPNP

Associate Professor of Pediatric Nursing
Yale University School of Nursing

and

Editor, *The Journal of School Nursing*

ABOUT THIS RESOURCE

This book aims to provide useful "Monday morning" strategies for the more common and the more difficult problems likely to be encountered by the school nurse. Its usefulness relies on a preexisting knowledge base of human illness and wellness. An objective framework is provided for identifying and managing health care issues among students and, to a lesser extent, school personnel. Checklists, charts, and suggested forms and form letters have been used liberally and may be reproduced for daily use. Parent letters are reproduced in Spanish.

School Nurse's Survival Guide is not a substitute for comprehensive texts on specific diseases. Not all topics likely to be encountered by the school nurse are covered. An attempt has been made to cover a variety of subjects in the area of physical and mental health; topics that lend themselves to straightforward management strategies have been selected. References are included for nurses, students, and sometimes for adults who are not health professionals.

With a greater emphasis on delivery of health services in schools, it is hoped that this book will serve as a practical guide to accomplishing more with the time and funds allotted to the school nurse, who is, after all, the backbone of school health.

Since useful techniques are "discovered" at the level of daily school nurse practice, the author invites reader comments.

Richard M. Adams, M.D.

CONTENTS

Chapter 3. Developmental and Emotional Problems of Elementary Students 51

Diagnosis of Mental Disorders (52)   The Mind-Body Dilemma (53)   School
Readiness and Developmental Screening (54)   Child Neglect or Abuse (55)
Mental Retardation and Slow Learners (55)   Learning Disabilities (56)
Attention Deficit Hyperactivity Disorder (ADHD) (56)   Psychosomatic
Complaints (57)   Conduct Disorder (58)   Classroom Management Strategies
(59)   Other Developmental Disorders (60)   Summary (61)   References (63)

Chapter 4. Behavioral and Emotional Problems of Adolescents 69

Getting Inside the Adolescent's Head (71)   Anxiety Disorders (72)   Eating
Disorders (74)   Depression (76)   Suicide (78)   Antisocial Behavior and
Violence (80)   Drug Abuse (82)   Psychotherapy (83)   School Nurse Role (84)
Summary (85)   References (86)

Chapter 5. Gay and Lesbian Youth 95

Real Stories (96)   From Kinsey to the Present (96)   What Caused Him to
Be Gay or Her to Be Lesbian? (97)   How Many Are There? (97)   Deviant Sex-
ual Behavior (97)   Sorting Through the Terminology Maze (99)   The Coming-
Out Process (100)   Counseling Gay and Lesbian Youth (100)   Telling Parents
and Others (102)   When Things Aren't Going Well (102)   Selling Self (103)
Well Families and Sick Families (104)   Keeping a Journal (104)   Review of
Strategies (105)   Final Thoughts (105)   Summary (106)   References (107)

Chapter 12.   Legal Frameworks for School Health 269

Chapter 13.   High-Risk Youth 295

Chapter 14.   School Health: The Next Decade 325

Epilogue 353

CHAPTER 1

ORGANIZING YOUR PROGRAM

Looking at Needs
Setting Priorities
Implementation
Opening a New School Clinic
Assessing Effectiveness
Additional Considerations
Summary
References
Chapter 1 Figures:

Chapter 1

ORGANIZING YOUR PROGRAM

Any provider of a service who is to maintain relevance must know the consumer.

—*Business axiom*

The primary mission of school health services is to remove health barriers to learning. At first glance this may seem a narrow focus to those health professionals concerned with the "whole child," but consider that any child in less than optimal health will usually perform below his or her potential in school. Thus, all health issues impacting students are legitimate areas of focus for school health professionals. Health and learning are symbiotic twins—when one falters, the other follows. School nurses are essential players not only in removing health barriers to learning but also in removing learning barriers to health.

Successful programs also rely heavily on the cooperation of parents, teachers, and community health agencies; consequently, this chapter will take a macro, or communitywide, approach to planning and managing school health services.

LOOKING AT NEEDS

The business world has long understood the axiom, "Know the customer." Any provider of a product or service who is to maintain relevance and survive must observe it. But who is the customer in school health? The student is, obviously, but there are others: parents, teachers, administrators, and community health professionals. You need to survey all these groups in the initial stages of formulating a program. Whether you are developing local school or districtwide health services, this essential first step must be accomplished with thoroughness. You may have to use written surveys because of the number of "clients" or "customers," but you can always add a personal touch with individual interviews. Talk to student council and PTA presidents and attend one of their meetings. Walk them through the survey explaining what information is needed. Combine open-ended and structured input. Open-ended questions project an attitude of wanting to know their needs. Figure 1-1, which is located at the end of this chapter, is a sample questionnaire for PTA presidents. It could also be used for student council members, even at the elementary level (with some revision and more verbal explanation).

If your school or school district is developing a health program for the first time, the survey will need to be more comprehensive. For an existing program, ask the "customers" to rate existing services and name desired services not currently available. Be sure to do this step even though you may not be able to implement their requests because of budgetary, legal, or ethical constraints.

Other evidence of health needs comes from national and statewide figures on morbidity and mortality; however, these cannot substitute for local data. For example, if the incidence of drug abuse approaches zero in a community, it would not make sense to commit heavy resources to a drug prevention program.

Schoolwide or districtwide health needs assessments may be as simple as requesting a computer printout in districts with well-developed reporting procedures or as laborious as a year-long prospective manual tabulation of health problems.

Community data (extra-school district) may come from a variety of sources; however, the county health department is usually the best source of general health statistics. Mental health data are harder to obtain and will depend on local resources and reporting procedures. Mental Health and Mental Retardation (MHMR) offices are a good source, as are nonprofit mental health agencies serving children.

One approach to developing a local profile of health problems in children and youth involves collecting four categories of data.

1. Mortality data, divided into five subcategories: trauma and violent causes (motor vehicle accidents, homicides, suicides); malignancy; acute infections (e.g., meningitis, pneumonia); drug-related; and other.

2. Morbidity data: reportable diseases (primarily infections, i.e., STDs, HIV); injuries; and "new morbidities" such as attention deficit hyperactivity disorder (ADHD), drug and alcohol abuse, and teen pregnancy. Other categories will vary according to local conditions.

3. Chronic disorders: Appropriate subcategories include asthma, seizure disorders, diabetes, cystic fibrosis, cerebral palsy, handicapping conditions (vision, hearing), mental disorders, and other conditions with the potential for causing school absenteeism or underachievement.

4. Other conditions and information: Track the incidence of pediculosis, scabies, ringworm, dental problems, and nutritional problems. You may wish to collect additional data, depending on unique local conditions. For example, if lead exposure exists in your community, this will be an important part of your data.

SETTING PRIORITIES

Now that you've collected the raw data from multiple sources, look at it to see if there are any gaps. Are all consumer groups represented? (Don't forget the community providers to whom you will be referring students.) Are the data comprehensive or at least representative of the health problems likely to be encountered in your area? Compare them with state and national figures to see if you have overlooked any areas.

Next, review the list for those conditions that

- are most serious or potentially life threatening;
- interfere with learning;
- respond to intervention strategies;
- can be influenced by school personnel, and
- can be managed in a cost-efficient manner.

Those that score high on all five criteria will be the priorities to which you devote the most resources.

The development of goals and objectives should flow naturally from your identified priorities. To be useful they must be clear and specific. Ideally, the objectives will be measurable so that you can see whether you are reaching them. The following are examples of a goal, an objective, and an activity of a school health service program:

I. Reduce the incidence of health-related absenteeism by 10%.
   A. Achieve and maintain 99% immunization level for measles.
      1. Provide school-based immunization clinics in areas of nonavailability.

   Goals and objectives should
   - ensure access to community treatment resources
   - fill service gaps
   - ensure compliance with federal, state, and local requirements
   - meet locally documented student health needs
   - comply with community values
   - meet standards promulgated by professional organizations

Identifying a health problem for which there is no adequate local referral resource often creates a dilemma. Some health professionals suggest that a problem should not be identified if effective intervention cannot be achieved. Others contend that parents should know all their child's health problems and bear the ultimate responsibility for follow-up. The decision is a local one.

The following example gives a mission statement and ten goals for an entire school system:

To enhance the educational process through the removal of health barriers to learning and by promotion of an optimal level of wellness and environmental safety for students and employees.

1. Assign central and local campus health services personnel.
2. Provide selected materials, supplies, and equipment as needed.
3. Provide health appraisal of students to promote early referral of health problems.
4. Contribute to improving student achievement by reducing the incidence of health-related absences.
5. Identify and ameliorate health problems that impair learning.
6. Serve as interface between school district and health care community.
7. Consult with Personnel Department regarding employee health issues.
8. Cooperate with the departments of Special Education and Health Education in achieving common goals for students.
9. Consult with the Athletics and Physical Education Departments regarding health issues in sports.
10. Serve as a resource to administration in environmental health issues.

Each goal would, of course, be accompanied by objectives and specific activities to achieve them—all measurable.

The school functions as a part of a community; consequently, a school health program should be part of the community health care network. You must decide which functions can and should be performed by your school.

IMPLEMENTATION

A chart or schedule of activities, with time lines, is the simplest method for establishing an implementation plan. This will be a dynamic document, changing from year to year as priorities shift. The person responsible for completing an activity should be listed (usually the nurse or nurse assistant) along with the date for completion.

Other elements of the implementation plan include provisions for staff management (an organization chart, job descriptions, personnel evaluations), parental involvement (through PTA or other groups), and networking with community personnel (informal and formal agreements with local health care providers and agencies).

No implementation plan will succeed without careful attention to referral resources. Unless you have an extensive network of school-based clinics, community health professionals will be treating your students. Without intervention, identifying a health problem has not helped a student.

While specific referral resources (community clinics, hospitals, and medical specialists) may not be included in your implementation plan, establishing these links is one of the most important elements of an effective school health service program. Existing community health resources and the socioeconomic level of the child must be matched for each problem to be addressed. For example, a 5-year-old with strabismus might best be referred to a pediatric ophthalmologist, while an adult eye care specialist might be appropriate for a 17-year-old. Mental health resources for low-income adolescents are notoriously sparse in many areas, even larger cities. Physician specialist volunteers and volunteer groups can serve as substitutes. School-based clinics are becoming more common to reduce service deficiencies (see Chapter 14).

Most states have Early and Periodic Screening, Diagnosis, and Treatment Programs (EPSDT), funded federally through Title XIX-Medicaid. These programs have built-in "provider lists" of participating physicians who will see specific types of health problems. EPSDT can also be a revenue source for school health programs, with an average reimbursement of $25 to $45 per child screened. Specially certified individuals such as nurse practitioners or physician's assistants might serve as an in-house resource to perform the screenings.

Midyear assessment of progress toward goal completion is always a good idea. A shift in resources may prevent failure to meet a stated objective.

OPENING A NEW SCHOOL CLINIC

The physical space, equipment and supplies required for a school clinic will depend on the program to be implemented and its budget. Figure 1-2 lists minimum supplies and equipment. The cost of this equipment at press time was $6,800. Suggested floor plans for elementary and secondary school health rooms are illustrated in Figures 1-3 and 1-4. Make your initial selection of space and equipment allowing for the potential to upgrade in the future.

ASSESSING EFFECTIVENESS

A number of reasons exist for expending time and energy on the evaluation of school health services. Among the most important are

- identification of successful program elements
- identification of unsuccessful program elements (leading to modified efforts)
- documentation of cost-effectiveness.

At budget time, nothing is more gratifying than having the numbers to show you delivered what you promised at a reasonable cost. It is often an eye-opener to school board members and administrators to see that adequate school health services can be provided for under $50 per student per year.

While a universal plan for evaluating a school health program cannot be offered (because of local variables), the checklist in Figure 1-5 can serve as a starting point. Checking off goals that have been met may seem easy; however, some may be met only partially (say, 75%), and the reasons for incomplete fulfillment may be varied, difficult to identify, or not under the control of school personnel. For instance, if dental referrals have only a 25% completion rate (a not uncommon figure), the reason may be insufficient or inaccessible dental resources, lack of parent funds, low parent priority, or any number of other causes. Teasing these out and developing remedies constitute the challenge as well as a reason for having goals in the first place. While goals and objectives are generally developed for one-year time blocks, it is advisable to think two and three years ahead—a process known as *strategic planning*.

The spirit of strategic planning is to add a new dimension to long-range planning by projecting trends from existing demographic data on several fronts: economics, social issues, ethnicity of populations, and educational issues. This process, while not always precise, allows for the development of the relevant and realistic goals; without it, schools are apt to ignore signs of the need for change.

ADDITIONAL CONSIDERATIONS

Budgeting

Most of the cost of a school health service program is accounted for by personnel (80% to 90% for most programs). Knowing how many nurses, nurse aides, secretaries, and other personnel are required to achieve stated goals and objectives will cover approximately 85% of your program's cost. The number of health service personnel needed flows from the activities required to meet the objectives developed. If the health history and health appraisal or physical examination take the average school nurse 60 minutes per student and the nurse is responsible for 850 students (half of whom are to be screened per year), it would require 425 hours of the nurse's time per year. On the basis of a 40-hour week for 36 weeks, this would constitute 30% of the school nurse's time.

Equipment and supplies also evolve from required screening. Based on activities to be performed and budgeting constraints, a well-stocked clinic can be created from the list in Figure 2.

Familiarity with the local budgeting process is essential whether the amount involved is a few thousand or several million dollars. In some school districts, goals and objectives are directly linked to dollars, while in other districts the process is less rigid. Additionally, zero-based budgeting is the new wave of school finance. Either way, provisions should be made for unexpected contingencies.

Staff Qualifications

School nurses are the backbone of any school health service program. The higher the educational status of the nursing staff, the higher program quality will be. Many school districts are requiring bachelor level candidates and recruiting as many master's-level nurses as possible, with practitioner status the ultimate. The schools that can secure and retain nurses at the higher end of the educational spectrum will have a head start on a quality program.

Program Manager

The individual chosen to head up the school health services program is most often a nurse, sometimes a physician. Either should not only be technically knowledgeable but also have management skills. Non-health professionals do not usually prove to be effective health service leaders.

Staff Development

The increasingly rapid growth of medical information and technology requires that regular professional growth programs be planned for school health professionals. The half-life of a school nurse's knowledge base has been estimated at no more than five years. Program content will depend on the types of student health problems being seen by school nurses, as well as on available speakers and consultants.

Medical Consultants

Physician specialty consultants are needed for both individual students and development of state-of-the-art practices and procedures. They may volunteer or be paid.

Health Advisory Council

Community health professionals, school personnel, parents, and students should help oversee school health services. This may be a formal task force or council or a series of ad hoc committees for specific issues.

Health Counseling

Every health service activity should be viewed as an opportunity for health education or counseling, whether it be with students, faculty, staff, or parents. See Chapter 6 for further discussion of this topic.

Cooperation with Other Departments

To maximize effectiveness, health service personnel will need linkages with other school departments, with overlapping responsibilities. These include, but are not limited to, special education, health education, physical education, food services, and personnel. An example of such effective cooperation is in the management of obese students where the local school nurse, cafeteria manager, PE teacher, and health educator work with the parents and community physician to effect weight loss and improve self-image.

Evaluation of Personnel

Employee performance assessment is the subject of numerous publications—many dealing with health professionals. Relative to the school nurse, *School Nursing Practice: Roles & Standards* (National Association of School Nurses, 1993) is the "gold standard" for the development of job descriptions upon which all evaluations should be based.

A particularly difficult situation arises when a school health employee is suffering from a mental health disorder or substance abuse. Minimal literature exists on psychiatric disability. A mental health assessment performed by a psychiatrist or psychologist outside the school district is usually the best approach. Physical disabilities are easier to assess and relate to a job description (see Chapter 8).

Employees who are not performing to expectations must be counseled early in the school year and given specific suggestions, with time to improve before final evaluations are done.

Employee Health

While student health is the focus of most school health service programs, faculty and staff inevitably seek first aid and advice on other health matters from school nurses. Employee assistance programs (EAP) seeking to deal with stress, substance abuse, and excessive absenteeism will often ask school health professionals to participate in the management of troubled employees (see Chapter 8).

Risk Management

Departments of risk management are beginning to appear in larger school districts. Generally they carry out an umbrella function of reducing financial losses through safety education and prevention programs and management of workers' compensation cases, as well as securing cost-effective insurance coverage for buses and other high cost items.

Environmental Issues

Following the asbestos abatement regulations, media coverage of radon hazards, and Alar on apples, school personnel and parents have become more attuned to environmental health hazards. Some are merely nuisances (odorous paint vapors) while others bear more careful evaluation (use of pesticides in schools). A system of reporting from local school to central administration should be developed so that appropriate investigations can be carried out. The services of a consulting industrial hygienist or environmental health specialist may be needed. This will be expanded further in Chapter 10.

Legal Issues

New laws and increasing litigation dictate that school health professionals have a reliable source of legal consultation. You must, however, guard against discontinuing an activity clearly beneficial to students because of a merely theoretical legal liability.

Computerized Data

Whether centralized or campus based, the computerization of student health information will facilitate quality control, mandated reporting, and clinical research. The assistance of a programmer is desirable. Immunization data are the easiest with which to begin. Other data that lend themselves to computer storage and retrieval include vision and hearing screening results and individual student health problems. Keeping track of the incidence of asthma, diabetes, or pregnancies will assist in focusing available resources. Commercially available software exists for computerizing student health records; more information is in Chapter 14.

Public Relations and Politics

Individuals with scientific backgrounds, including health professionals, are often surprised and distressed to find that in the public sector decisions are not always made entirely on objective grounds. School health decisions may seem straightforward to the local school nurse who knows the medical facts but not the perceptions of the public or the personal philosophies of school trustees. For example, a decision to require tuberculosis clearance in students who are recent immigrants from countries having a high incidence of tuberculosis seems simple. However, since Mexico and numerous African countries are on this list, suspicions of racism may be expressed. Although entirely subjective and unfounded, they must be dealt with.

Sharing Ideas

Once a program is up and running, a good method of fine-tuning it is to share successes and unmet challenges with school districts of similar or larger size, particularly in the same state. "How we do it" sessions at seminars or annual conventions are good forums for this. Reading professional journals is also helpful.

SUMMARY

The key elements to implementing an effective (and cost-effective) school health service program are

- Comprehensive data on local health problems
- A prioritized list of health problems to be addressed
- A realistic and comprehensive set of goals and objectives
- Familiarity with the budgeting process
- A knowledgeable health professional manager
- Adequate networking with community health personnel
- Inclusion of parents and students at all levels
- Objective program and personnel evaluations
- Willingness to make program adjustments
- Knowledge of legal and ethical issues
- Attention to public relations and political issues
- Sharing of successes and challenges with other programs*

Each school health service program will be unique based upon local philosophy, needs, and resources. What each should share is a child-oriented focus that provides services based on identified student needs.

---

*Publication of an annual report is an ideal way to do this. See Figure 1-6, "Model Annual Report," for an example.

REFERENCES

1. Adams, R. M. "Planning and Management of School Health Services." In *Principles and Practices of Student Health,* Vol. 1, pp. 291–301. Oakland, CA: Third Party Publishing, 1991.

2. Earle, J. *How Schools Work and How to Work with Schools: A Guide for Health Professionals.* Alexandria, VA: National Association of State Boards of Education, 1990.

3. Kawamoto, Kristi. "Nursing Leadership: To Thrive in a World of Change." *Nursing Administration Quarterly* 18(3):1–6, 1994.

4. Nader, P. R. (ed.). "Organization & Staffing of School Health Services" in *School Health: Policy and Practice,* pp. 78–79. Elk Grove Village, IL: American Academy of Pediatrics, 1993.

5. Newton, J. *The New School Health Handbook.* Englewood Cliffs, NJ: Prentice Hall, 1989, pp. 1–15.

6. Proctor, S. T. *School Nursing Practice: Roles and Standards.* Scarborough, ME: National Association of School Nurses, 1993.

7. __. *School Nursing Practice: Roles and Standards.* Scarborough, ME: National Association of School Nurses, 1993.

8. Sullivan, E. *Effective Management in Nursing.* Redwood City, CA: Benjamin/Cummings Publishing, 1992.

9. Umiker, W. *Management Skills for the New Health Care Supervisor.* Rockville, MD: Aspen, 1988.

10. Woodfill, M. M. *The Role of the Nurse in the School Setting.* Kent, OH: American School Health Association, 1991.

Figure 1-1

SCHOOL HEALTH SERVICE QUESTIONNAIRE FOR PTA GROUPS

I. Major areas of School Health Service Activities:

Below is a list of student services offered by the _____ School District. Please check those activities you know to be available in your child's school.

_____ Health assessments, medical referrals, and follow-up

_____ Vision testing

_____ Hearing testing

_____ First aid

_____ Immunization review and referral

_____ Dental examination

_____ Height/weight measurement

_____ Administration of medication

_____ Special procedures (bladder catheterization, blood glucose monitoring, etc.)

_____ Limited or modified physical education

_____ Teacher/nurse conferences for program adjustments pertinent to health problems

_____ Staffing conference for student placement in special learning situations

_____ Health education

_____ Individual health counseling

_____ Home visits

_____ Other (please explain) _____

_____

II. Please list the current School Health Services activities that you feel are adequate:

_____

_____

_____

III. List current School Health Services activities that could be improved:

_____

_____

_____

Figure 1-1 *(Continued)*

IV. Please list those services that are not currently available but would be desirable:

_____

_____

_____

V. What PTA activities do you feel are currently being adequately coordinated with the school nurse?

_____ Nurse participation in PTA activities

_____ Nurse cooperation with PTA health chairperson

_____ Preschool Round-up (elementary level)

_____ Transportation for students with health problems

_____ Parent health room volunteers

_____ Other (explain)

VI. What PTA activities do you feel warrant more attention and cooperation from the local building nurse and/or from central School Health Service staff?

_____

_____

_____

VII. Are you acquainted with the current Red Cross Health Room Volunteer Program?

_____ Yes

_____ No

If yes, please express your feeling about the adequacy of that project:

_____

_____

_____

VIII. Additional Comments: _____

_____

_____

ENCUESTA DE SERVICIOS ESCOLARES DE SALUD PARA PADRES Y MIEMBROS DE LA PTA

I. Actividades principales en las áreas de Servicios Escolares de Salud:

A continuación tenemos una lista de servicios para estudiantes ofrecidos por el Distrito

Escolar de _____. Por favor, marque las actividades que se ofrecen en la escuela de su hijo/a.

_____ Evaluación de salud, referidos médicos, y continuación de servicios

_____ Pruebas de la vista

_____ Pruebas de audición

_____ Primeros auxilios

_____ Revisión de las vacunas y referidos médicos

_____ Pruebas dentales

_____ Medidas de peso/estatura

_____ Administración de medicinas

_____ Procedimientos especiales (caterización de le vejiga, verificar niveles de glucosa)

_____ Educación física limitada o modificada

_____ Conferencias de maestra/enfermera para ajustes pertinentes a los problemas de salud.

_____ Conferencias con empleados para colocar al estudiante en situaciones especiales de aprendizaje.

_____ Instrucción sobre la salud

_____ Consejería individual sobre la salud

_____ Visitas al hogar

_____ Otra (por favor explíque) _____

_____

II. Mencione los Servicios Escolares de Salud y actividades que usted cree son aceptables:

_____

_____

_____

III. Mencione los Servicios Escolares de Salud que pueden ser mejorados:

_____

_____

IV. Mencione los servicios que al momento no existen en su escuela, pero que desearía tenerlos:

_____

_____

_____

V. ¿Cuáles actividades de la PTA usted cree son coordinadas adecuadamente con la enfermera de la escuela?

_____ Participación de la enfermera en actividades de la PTA

_____ Cooperación de la enfermera con la representante del área de salud de la PTA

_____ Matrícula a nivel pre-escolar (nivel primaria)

_____ Transportación para estudiantes con problemas de salud

_____ Participación de padres como voluntarios en las clases de Educación de la Salud

_____ Otro (explique)

VI. ¿Qué actividades de la PTA usted cree necesitan más atención y cooperación por parte de la enfermera de la escuela y/o el personal de la administración de Servicios Escolares de Salud?

_____

_____

_____

VII. ¿Tiene usted conocimiento sobre el Programa de Voluntarios en la Clase De Salud de la Cruz Roja?

_____ Sí

_____ No

Si respondió "Sí," por favor exprese su opinión si ese programa fué suficiente:

_____

_____

_____

_____

VIII. Comentarios Adicionales: _____

_____

_____

_____

Figure 1-2

SUGGESTED ITEMS FOR OPENING A NEW SCHOOL CLINIC

Furniture
- Desk
- Secretarial chair
- Two-drawer filing cabinet
- Revolving stool
- Small refrigerator
- Stainless steel utility cart
- Gooseneck examination lamp
- Waste receptacles (2)

Major Medical Equipment
- Examination table
- Recovery couch with paper rolls (4)
- Scales with height bar
- Wheelchair (optional)
- Stretcher
- Audiometer
- Diagnostic set (oto-ophthalmoscope)

Minor Medical Equipment
- Occluders for vision test
- Pocket aneroid blood pressure set, adult size
- Pocket aneroid blood pressure set, child size
- Stethoscopes (2)
- Glass sundry jar set (with rack)
- *Physicians' Desk Reference (PDR)*
- Medical dictionary
- Plus Lens, 3.0 glasses (1 pair)
- Emesis basins (2)
- Cotton blankets (6)
- Tackle boxes (for portable supplies) (2)
- Heating pads (2)
- Penlights (2)
- Measuring tape
- Percussion hammer
- Tweezers/pick-ups (3)
- Instrument tray (2)
- 20-foot Snellen Vision Chart
- HOTV Vision Chart
- Color vision test: 10-plate Ishihara for pre-readers (optional)

Supplies
- Examination paper (12 rolls)
- Cold compresses (4, freezable)
- Cotton balls (2 packages)
- Drinking cups (6 boxes)
- Tongue depressors (4 boxes)
- Gauze pads (4 packages)
- Stretch gauze (2)
- Gloves, size medium (4 boxes of 100 pairs)*
- Ipecac (2 bottles, 4 fluid ounces each)
- Bar soap, or liquid soap with dispenser (20 bars)
- Adhesive tape (1/2 inch) (20 rolls)
- Oral thermometers (6 dozen)
- Cotton-tipped applicators (20 packages of 100)
- Vaseline, plain (12)
- Band-aids (20 boxes of 30)
- Wescodyne (2 gallons) (or comparable disinfectant suitable for thermometers)

*Universal precaution procedures require gloves to be worn for all first aid and emergency procedures involving blood.

Figure 1-3

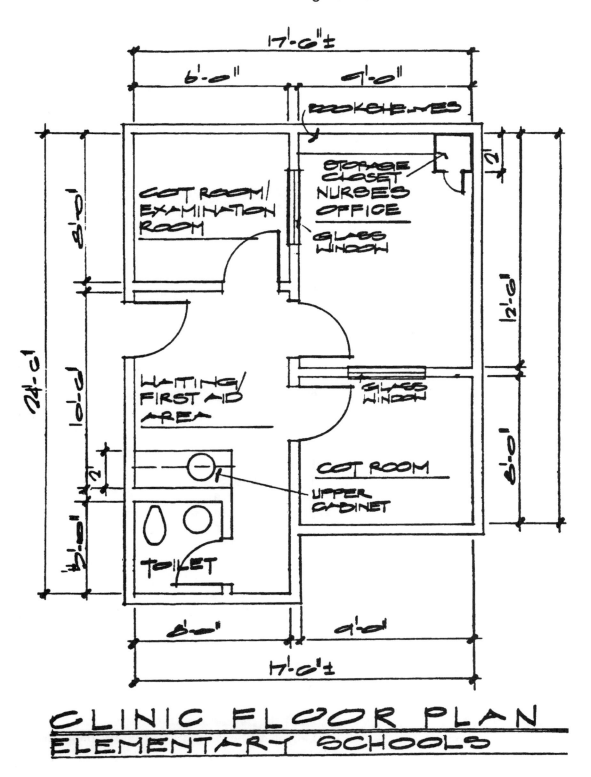

CLINIC FLOOR PLAN
ELEMENTARY SCHOOLS

Figure 1-4

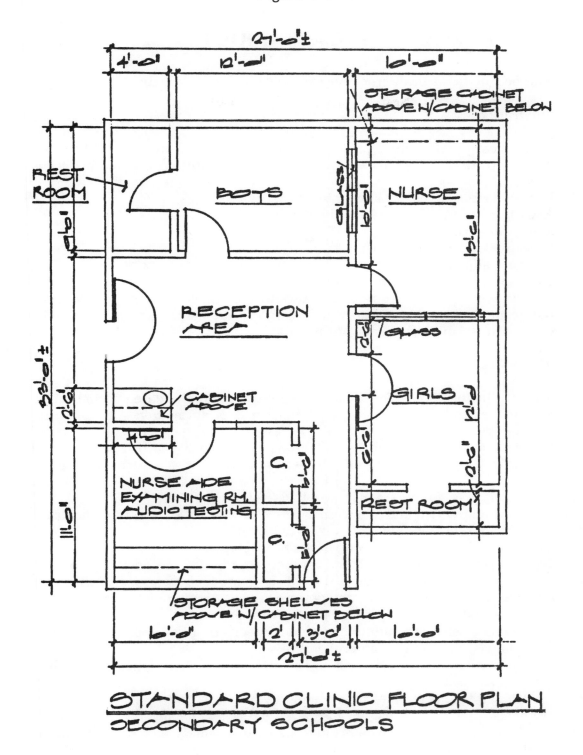

STANDARD CLINIC FLOOR PLAN
SECONDARY SCHOOLS

Figure 1-5

PLAN FOR EVALUATING A SCHOOL HEALTH PROGRAM

Items should be rated on a scale from one (not met) to five (fulfilled):

I. Administration

   A. School board philosophy and policies provide for an effective school health program.
   B. Administrative guidelines facilitate the implementation of effective school health services.
   C. Budgetary resources are adequate.
   D. Activities and services are based on student need.
   E. Measurable goals are set.
   F. Objective evaluation is performed.
   G. Program adjustments are made based on evaluation results.
   H. Legal standards of health care are met.
   I. The student:school nurse ratio is determined by student health needs, legal requirements, number of individuals with special health care needs, mobility of population, and other relevant factors.

II. Health Services

   A. A health history is obtained on entering students and updated periodically.
   B. A health appraisal or physical examination is performed on entering students and updated periodically.
   C. Selected screening procedures are performed to identify health barriers to learning.
   D. Immunization monitoring and other communicable disease control programs are in place.
   E. Provisions exist for emergency care and first aid.
   F. Appropriate referral and follow-up care are carried out on identified health problems.
   G. Effective parent communication is established.
   H. Networking with community agencies is developed.
   I. Technical currency is maintained through appropriate staff development.
   J. School personnel are encouraged to observe students for possible health problems and are given in-service training on recognizing such problems or emergencies.
   K. Ethical standards of health care practice are met.
   L. Provisions exist for the administration of medication and special procedures.
   M. Child abuse reporting is comprehensive.
   N. Health services personnel recommend necessary school adjustments for students with health problems.
   O. Health services personnel make home or hospital visits related to student health problems.
   P. Accidents are analyzed to determine their cause; safety hazards are reported.
   Q. Health services personnel assist in special educational placement and provide designated nursing services.
   R. Health services personnel assist families in obtaining free or partial-pay health services when necessary.
   S. Clinical research is conducted to determine efficacy of activities and procedures (optional).
   T. An annual report is prepared.

Figure 1-5 *(Continued)*

III. Health Education

    A. Health services personnel cooperate with other school professionals to meet formal and informal health education goals.

    B. Health service personnel serve as consultants to health educators.

    C. All health service activities are utilized as teaching/learning opportunities.

    D. Health services personnel conduct programs for parent-teacher organizations and community groups.

IV. School Environment

    A. The district provides a physical plant and equipment that meet the educational needs of its students and staff.

    B. School health personnel assume shared responsibility for the safety and comfort of the school environment.

    C. Mechanisms exist for addressing potential environmental health hazards.

    D. Safety education and injury prevention are given high priority.

    E. Federal, state, and local regulations on environmental safety are observed.

    F. A smoke-free environment is provided.

    G. Fire and disaster plans are established.

    H. The school lunch program is utilized as a learning laboratory for good nutrition.

(Adapted from the Texas Education Agency)

Figure 1-6

MODEL ANNUAL REPORT
(SUMMARY PAGE)

Clinic Visits

Student

Illness/Health Maintenance	449,546
Minor Trauma	106,030
Major Trauma	307
Other Student Visits	180,561
Total Student Visits	736,444

Adult

Employees	23,944
Other Adults	107,212
Total Adult Visits	131,156
GRAND TOTAL CLINIC VISITS	867,600

Enrollment	=	139,819
Clinic visits per student/year	=	5.3

Health Screening	Screened	Referred		Completed	
Health Appraisal	41,453	968	(2.3%)	331	(34.0%)
Dental	40,942	6,268	(15.0%)	1,231	(20.0%)
Vision	82,542	5,401	(7.0%)	2,776	(51.0%)
Hearing	69,444	3,011	(4.3%)	1,715	(57.0%)
Spinal Screening (5, 8)	17,596	260	(1.47%)	54	(20.7%)

Complete History and Physical Examination (In-house)

EPSDT (Title XIX)	268
Special Education	276
Health Maintenance	109
Total Physical Examinations	653

Immunization Protection Levels (%)

Measles #1	99.5
Measles #2	99.5
Mumps	99.4
Rubella	99.6
Polio	99.0
Diphtheria/Tetanus	98.6
HIB	93.4
Average Compliance Level	98.4%

Figure 1-6 (Continued)

Pediculosis

Student cases identified and treated	5,889	>20,215
Family members treated	14,326	
Cost of pediculicide	$71,763.00	
Cost per treatment	$ 3.55	

Child Abuse: 389 cases reported

Cost Analysis

1992–93 Health Services Central Budget . . . .$ 206,623.00
Nurse Salaries 3,963,501.00
Nurse Aide/Assistant Salaries 1,042,384.00
Total Expenditure 5,212,508.00

Enrollment 139,818.00

Per Pupil Expenditure/Year . . . .$ 37.28

CHAPTER 2

CHRONIC PHYSICAL PROBLEMS

Chapter 2

CHRONIC PHYSICAL PROBLEMS

A ship in harbor is safe—but that is not what ships are for.

John A. Shedd

About 15% of children have some chronic health condition. Most of those are mild and have little effect on school attendance or performance. However, 2% to 4% of school-age children have severe chronic illnesses that routinely disrupt school participation.

As recently as the 1970s, almost half of these severely affected children died before graduation age. Now, 80% to 90% achieve graduation thanks to better medical care. Such children frequently require special procedures and technological support to participate in school. School nurses enable schools to serve chronically disabled students educationally without undue concern for their physical well being.

This chapter will review the scope of physical conditions and procedures faced by school nurses in the 1990s and beyond. The guiding principle for all health and educational efforts is "normalization" to the extent possible.

THE TOP TEN

A chronic physical problem is defined as an anatomical or chemical abnormality that interferes with the normal functioning of a young person.

Figure 2-1, at the end of this chapter, illustrates the ten most common chronic physical disorders in a large urban school district. Asthma is the leader by far and is the only childhood condition for which the death rate is increasing. This alarming fact in the face of advanced treatment methods warrants the use of asthma as a paradigm for the management of chronic physical disorders.

Conditions in positions two through ten are epilepsy, hearing loss, visual impairment, scoliosis, cerebral palsy, sickle cell disease, diabetes, congenital heart disease and malignancy. Any of these could as easily be used as the model for service delivery to chronically disabled students.

SERVICE DELIVERY MODELS

Regina is an 11-year-old newly enrolled student with moderately severe asthma who, although capable, misses three to four days of school per month—more during winter. She is shy and superficially cooperative with the school nurse. Regina's mother minimizes the seriousness of her daughter's asthma suggesting "it's mostly in her head." Teachers are frustrated with the constant need to provide make-up work, although they do so because of Regina's potential. The school nurse is at the school three days per week and notes that Regina does not always come in for her medication on the other two days.

Faced with this challenge the school nurse implements the following steps:

1. Initial health history completed by Regina's mother (Figure 2-2).
2. Physician Questionnaire and Request for Administration of Medicine (Figures 2-3 and 2-4) sent to family doctor.
3. Regina's Individualized Health Plan recorded for her teachers (Figure 2-5).
4. Above information shared with classroom teachers along with generic health information for the child with asthma (Figure 2-6).
5. Emergency telephone numbers for mother and physician recorded in Regina's file.

Further conversations with the physician and mother resulted in an evaluation by an asthma specialist that revealed multiple allergies to pollens and molds. The specialist began hyposensitization and recommended further maternal counseling with the school nurse regarding the physical nature of Regina's problems (stress did not seem to precipitate wheezing) and the importance of regular medication even when Regina felt well. The mother became more supportive and Regina showed progress toward self-direction. She even gave a report to her classes on her asthma and its control.

The school nurse also identified issues to be addressed in the future:

• Has attendance improved?
• Has academic performance improved?
• Is Regina ready to assume responsibility for taking her medication?
• Are there lingering psychological or social problems?

Consideration for special education services was unnecessary for Regina.

MEDICALLY FRAGILE STUDENTS

A medically fragile child is one who has a life-threatening condition and requires the oversight of a skilled professional nurse. These students may require schedule adjustments and frequent visits to the doctor as well as daily medication and special procedures. Examples are students with malignancies, sickle cell disease, or AIDS. Figure 2-7 lists special procedures that may be required at school. Because most procedures take only a few minutes and full-time nurse coverage is the exception, health aides may be trained to do them. The purchase of equipment and supplies varies from state to state, but generally parents are expected to furnish expendable supplies such as catheters, suction tips, and diapers.

One of the first decisions to be made regarding a child with a chronic physical condition is whether he or she should be placed in a special education class. The primary consideration should be cognitive ability. When feasible a student should be placed in regular education classes (accessibility should not be an issue as schools have the responsibility of removing physical barriers to "mainstreaming"). As well, the flexibility of current federal legislation allows for regular education class placement with special education support services. Examples of such services include occupational or speech therapy and transportation. In borderline cases, a child should receive a trial placement in regular class, because once special education placement is made movement in the other direction is less likely.

PHYSICAL EDUCATION

Physical fitness (including cardiovascular) is important for all individuals, but of special importance for the physically handicapped child. With few exceptions, some form of adapted physical education can be devised for physically challenged students. Some schools have adaptive PE specialists who can, with the school nurse's help, take the physical restrictions imposed by the physician and develop a modified physical education or fitness program for most students.

Participation in PE class, when possible, has obvious benefits beyond fitness. It enhances socialization and self-esteem. Far too many children are exempted from PE participation for fear of merely theoretical problems or legal liability. These can be avoided when parents, physician, and school plan together.

WHO PERFORMS PROCEDURES?

Ideally a school nurse should perform, or at least oversee, all procedures. The lack of full-time nurse coverage, however, requires others to be involved. With physician and parent permission and proper training, health aides, teachers, and teacher aides can perform most procedures required at school (with periodic RN monitoring). A good rule of thumb is: If the parent performs the procedure at home, a non-health professional can do it at school. One example is bladder catheterization.

When non-health professionals are expected to carry out medical procedures, it should be written into their job descriptions: "Special education teacher aides will perform selected health procedures with nurse training and supervision. Such procedures may include, but are not limited to, bladder catheterization, gastrostomy feeding, and intestinal ostomy care."

Perhaps the most demanding procedure is tracheotomy suctioning. Not only must proper technique be observed, but emergencies must be anticipated and handled competently, such as changing a blocked tracheotomy tube. Some non-health paraprofessionals may not be able to adjust psychologically to such responsibility and should not be forced to assume it against their will.

GIVING MEDICATION TO UNCOOPERATIVE STUDENTS

Uncooperative students are those who either willfully, or due to lack of adequate swallowing, are a challenge to give medication to. The drugs prescribed for disabled students are essential for their well-being and missed doses—for example, anticonvulsants—may have serious consequences. Gilda Landreneau of Shreveport, Louisiana, has this to say on the subject:

> Liquid meds are especially difficult to give in children with poor swallowing and those determined not to take it. An unpleasant taste compounds the problem. Pills are easier to give because they can be "sneaked in" with food. Capsules can be opened and the powder added to food. (This may not apply to certain timed-release capsules—check with the prescribing physician or pharmacist.) Large tablets can be crushed, preferably with a mortar and pestle; otherwise, you may lose some. If all else fails, another route of administration might be chosen by the doctor (suppository, injection, or dermal patch).

TRANSPORTATION

The influx to public schools of students with complex disabilities has created the need for more sophisticated transportation. Although the school bus may still be short and yellow, the similarity ends there. Special education or "handicap buses" now are being seen with these additions:

- wheelchair lifts
- air conditioning
- seat belts and child safety seats
- emergency equipment (suction machines, etc.)

- trained bus drivers
- bus monitors
- two-way radios

Approximately 400,000 school buses are used to transport 25 million school children four billion miles each year in the United States (National Research Council, 1989). Fifteen percent of these carry 15 or fewer passengers and are mostly for handicapped students. The school bus safety record is considerably better than that for private vehicles: Of the approximately 150 people killed in school bus accidents each year, only 12% are passengers.

Transportation of preschool-age disabled children is a particular challenge and more likely to require a trained adult monitor in addition to the driver. Combining the need for restraint with proper positioning for the individual child requires special attention and creativity.

For older, less physically disabled students, compartmentalization is a viable option. This means keeping passengers confined to a padded compartment as crash protection. It includes high padded setbacks and small distances between seat rows. Some authorities feel this option is preferable to seat belts because of the low utilization rate of the latter.

Radial tires and antilock brake systems are also gaining popularity, but the most important safety device on a school bus is a trained driver. The American Academy of Pediatrics makes the following recommendations for school bus driver selection and training (1993):

1. Maintain a valid commercial driver's license.
2. Be a minimum of 21 years of age.
3. Show proof of a yearly health examination, including vision and hearing.
4. Maintain a satisfactory driving record and successfully pass a criminal record check.
5. Attend a minimum of 6 hours of instruction including: (a) emergency and accident-related procedures; (b) first aid; (c) basic knowledge of the developmental stages and the needs of school-age children; (d) transportation of special needs pupils.
6. Successfully complete a written or oral test covering topics described in recommendation 5, as well as a driving performance test, and demonstrate safe loading and unloading procedures.
7. Submit to mandatory drug testing.

While transportation and special education officials may be responsible for designing school bus procedures for disabled students, you can serve an essential role by making weekly spot checks before a bus driver leaves the school campus at the end of the day. As school nurse, you are in the best position to know the needs and precautions for individual children.

HOSPITAL OR HOME INSTRUCTION

Schools are required by law to provide hospital or home instruction as an option for students. Generally such instruction is for students who will be absent from school for a minimum of two to four weeks. Sometimes greater flexibility is provided for multiple short absences as in children with hemophilia or sickle cell disease. Written physician statements are usually required for entry to and exit from hospital or homebound instruction. Figures 2-8 and 2-9 illustrate sample forms for this purpose. The school nurse may need to interpret or obtain clarification of these physician statements.

Parents of homebound students have a responsibility to provide a proper setting for learning that includes a responsible adult in the house (but not in the room) during classes. The student should be ready for work when the teacher arrives. A call should be made to the teacher if the student is unable to have class or if anyone in the home has an infectious disease.

CASE MANAGEMENT

If the overall case manager for a given handicapped child is someone other than the school nurse, the nurse still retains primary responsibility for supervision and management of health issues. This should not prove problematic when transdisciplinary cooperation is in place. The school nurse is always the most appropriate link with community physicians and health agencies. You best understand the priorities of health care issues and the necessity for anticipating future needs, including possible emergencies. Nurses are especially important when a child has no medical home, but are no less important when multiple specialty providers are involved with a single child (so the right hand knows what the left hand is doing).

Attendance at pupil personnel committee meetings can be time consuming, but it is time well spent to get things off on the right track. All allied health professionals have an important contribution to make, but when dealing with physically disabled students, the occupational therapist (OT) is especially helpful. When you are faced with problems of feeding and other activities of daily living, the OT is a strong ally in developing comprehensive care plans. Other areas to which OTs contribute include mobility, assistive devices, transfers, bypass techniques, and parent training and support.

OTs may evaluate a student upon a nurse's request. In many states, any form of therapy requires a physician prescription or order. The therapy program can be spelled out by the OT, then signed by the doctor (sometimes after changes are made).

It is self-evident that good school health records are essential to adequate monitoring and follow-through, to say nothing of potential legal usefulness.

EFFECTS OF CHRONIC ILLNESS ON THE FAMILY

Ideally, the majority of family interactions are positive and reinforcing to its members. But, even in the best of families, a disabled child induces stress. The following factors are most often responsible for stress in parents and other family members:

- cost
- daily burden of child care
- uncertainty of prognosis
- need for multiple providers and appointments
- effect on siblings
- marital conflict

The child with terminal illness is the most taxing scenario for parents and professionals. Experience has taught us that there is no facile or comfortable way to deal with the probability of death. It's a difficult business and it never gets easier. The school nurse who recognizes and deals with the reality of dying in a forthright manner does the affected child and parents an invaluable service, and exemplifies the marriage of art and science in health care. Dealing with teachers and other students is also an important part of this management challenge. Often this requires the involvement of the school psychologist, or other counselor, as well as community professionals.

Don't be too quick, however, to turn a student case over to a school psychologist; a new professional in the picture may merely add to parental stress. Rather, you may best use the psychologist as a consultant and select those recommendations that best suit a particular family's needs.

GENERAL PRINCIPLES

The policy statement of the National Association of School Nurses, "The School Nurse and the Student with Special Health Needs," provides a good summary of the school nurse's role in caring for students with chronic, disabling conditions:

> The National Association of School Nurses endorses the philosophy underlying P.L. 94-142, the Education of Handicapped Children Act.* This legislation guarantees the availability of free, appropriate public education for all children with special health needs in the least restrictive environment. Students with special health needs may require additional educational services as well as related health services.

---

*Current legislation is referred to as IDEA (Individuals with Disabilities Education Act).

The school nurse as a member of the evaluation team:

1. Assists in identifying candidates for placement in a special program.
2. Conducts the initial health evaluation and parent conference.
3. Obtains an in-depth health and developmental history and home environment assessment.
4. Provides and interprets all pertinent medical information, including results of recent physical assessments.
5. Develops the Individual Health Plan (IHP) with parent.
6. Provides the evaluation team with the health component for the Individual Educational Plan (IEP).
7. Confers with student, parent, and faculty to revise the health maintenance plan as needed.
8. Assists parent and student to use appropriate community resources.
9. Follows up on medical recommendations and reports to teachers and appropriate personnel.
10. Provides teacher/staff in-service regarding health maintenance plan of student.
11. Provides and/or supervises nursing treatment and specialized health procedures to allow the student to remain in the least restrictive environment.
12. Provides support to teacher, parent, and students who have specialized health care needs.

COVERING ALL THE BASES

Review and modification of a student's total management plan can be simplified by considering five major categories: medical, environmental, developmental, social, and educational. The child's developmental stage and skills plus his or her social context at home and school will often dictate the desired physical environment and method of delivery for medical services. For example, children with cerebral palsy or spina bifida often vary widely in their motor, cognitive, language and psychosocial skills. Cookbook plans will not get the job done—at least not in an optimum fashion for the child. Each area must be considered separately. A student who does not understand his or her medical condition or the reason for the medical procedures cannot be treated the same as one who does. Thus, INDIVIDUALIZED HEALTH PLAN (IHP)—with emphasis on the *I*.

The guiding principles in serving students with disabilities are to maximize

- school attendance and performance
- health management (including self-direction when appropriate)

- mental health (including socialization and self-esteem).
- career opportunities.

KEEPING UP WITH TECHNOLOGY

Keeping up with new technology requires vigilance, but the effort is essential; it pays dividends to students and conserves nurse time.

Peak Flow Meter

Providing adequate care in the school setting means staying abreast of new developments in health management. In our opening example of Regina's asthma, adequate care would include periodic monitoring of breathing efficiency with a peak flow meter. While the parents should have one at home, schools will find it advantageous to have one in each clinic. Disposable cardboard mouth pieces allow one instrument to be used for several students. The cost is minimal and you can determine much earlier when a student with asthma is approaching respiratory failure (long before cyanosis is present).

Glucometer

The glucometer, another valuable technology, monitors blood sugar in students with diabetes. It provides readings that are more accurate than those obtained using Dextrostix. It also allows testing by non-health professionals who lack the nurse's clinical judgment. And, of course, students of seven years and older can usually perform the test themselves.

Water-Pik for Earwax Removal

For unknown reasons, many students with handicaps accumulate cerumen in the external auditory canals. Retarded students are particularly prone to cerumenal impaction, which can reduce hearing.

A simple and safe method for removing earwax that occludes the auditory canal involves instilling mineral oil in the ear for a few days followed by irrigation with a Water-Pik. The details are:

1. Examine the ear canal with an otoscope to determine the extent of occlusion with cerumen.
2. Instill two to three drops of mineral oil in the affected ear(s) twice daily for three days.

3. Examine the ear canal with an otoscope to determine if occlusion is still present (sometimes the mineral oil alone clears the canal).

4. The patient's ear canal is straightened by pulling back and up on the ear. Direct the stream of water from the Water-Pik tip against the wall of the ear canal. *It is critically important to use a low setting* (no greater than ¼ of maximum). The water used should be lukewarm (about body temperature).

5. Reexamine ear. If it is still not clear, repeat steps 1 to 4.

BORDERLAND BETWEEN PHYSICAL AND MENTAL HEALTH

As science advances, the line between physical and mental problems blurs. Epilepsy, for example, sometimes produces cognitive and behavioral problems. Evidence is mounting to strongly suggest that disorders formerly thought to be purely "mental" represent chemical imbalances (e.g., manic-depressive disorder—now called bipolar disorder). Further, physical disorders frequently produce secondary emotional problems. These observations force us to conclude that separation of mind and body is neither possible nor desirable.

The next chapter will deal with those disorders that have predominantly mental manifestations in elementary students.

SUMMARY

In serving students with chronic physical handicaps, you must strike a balance between the "standard treatment plan" for a given problem and individual needs. Each student requires a slightly different twist for ideal management. What that twist should be is determined through sound professional judgment—flexible and creative professional judgment. Student, parent, and teacher personalities must always be taken into consideration.

One of the best tests for quality of care remains, "What would I want for my own child?"

REFERENCES

1. Haas, M. B. *The School Nurse's Source Book of Individualized Health Care Plans.* North Branch, MN: Sunrise River Press, 1993.

2. Hobbs, N. (ed.). *Issues in the Care of Children with Chronic Illness.* San Francisco: Jossey-Bass, 1985.

3. Jessop, D. J. "Providing Comprehensive Health Care to Children with Chronic Illnesses." *Pediatrics* 93 (4):602–607, 1994.

4. Nader, P. R. (ed.). "Children with Chronic Illness." In *School Health: Policy and Practice.* Elk Grove Village, IL: American Academy of Pediatrics, 1993, pp. 188–195.

5. —. "Technology-Supported Students." In *School Health,* pp. 196–205.

6. Newton, Jerry. *The New School Health Handbook.* Englewood Cliffs, NJ: Prentice Hall, 1989.

7. Passarelli, C. "Case Management of Chronic Health Conditions of School-Age Youth." In *Principles and Practices of Student Health,* Vol. 2, pp. 350–359. Oakland, CA: Third Party Publishing, 1992.

8. Pearl, L. M. "Training Competencies for School Health Professionals Working with Handicapped Children." *Journal of School Health* 58(7):298–300, 1988.

9. "Provision of Related Services for Children with Chronic Disabilities." (American Academy of Pediatrics, Position Statement of the Committee on Children with Disabilities.) *Pediatrics* 92(6):879–881, 1993.

10. "Psychosocial Risks of Chronic Health Conditions in Childhood and Adolescence." (American Academy of Pediatrics, Position Statement of the Committee on Children with Disabilities and the Committee on Psychosocial Aspects of Child and Family Health.) *Pediatrics* 92(6):876–77, 1993.

11. "Qualifications and Utilization of Nursing Personnel Delivering Health Services in Schools." *Pediatrics* 78(4):647–48, 1987.

12. "School Bus Transportation of Children with Special Needs." (American Academy of Pediatrics, Position Statement of the Committee on Injury and Poison Prevention.) *Pediatrics* 93(1):129–130, 1994.

13. Sternberg, Les. *Educating Students with Severe or Profound Handicaps.* Rockville, MD: Aspen, 1988.

14. *The Medically Fragile Child in the School Setting.* Washington, DC: American Federation of Teachers, 1992.

15. Walker, D. K. "Children and Youth with Special Health Care Needs." In *Principles and Practices of Student Health,* Vol. 1, pp. 185–194. Oakland, CA: Third Party Publishing, 1992.

16. Wood, S. P. "School Health Practices for Children with Complex Medical Needs." *Journal of School Health* 56(6):217–17, 1986.

Figure 2-1

TOP TEN CHRONIC PHYSICAL PROBLEMS
IN AN URBAN SCHOOL DISTRICT

(Enrollment = 140,000)

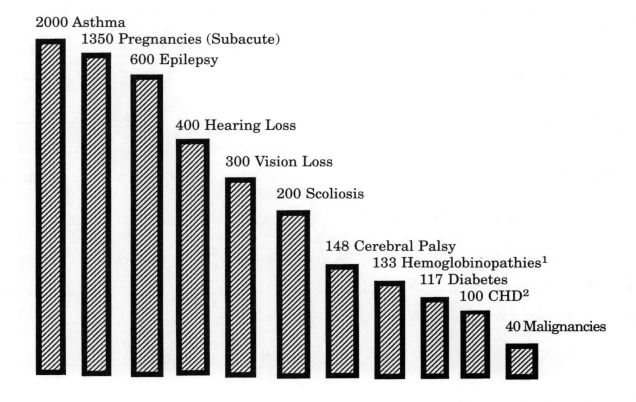

[1]Sickle cell trait/disease, etc. (African American Enrollment = 44%)
[2]Congenital Heart Disease

Figure 2-2

SCHOOL HEALTH SERVICE
HEALTH HISTORY

_____
School

_____
Grade

Dear Parent:

We would like your child to gain the most from his/her school experience. In order for us to assist in accomplishing this, it is necessary to have a current health history. Please complete this form and return it to the principal or nurse.

YOUR SCHOOL NURSE

Pupil's Name _____ Sex _____ Birth Date _____
       Last   First   Middle

Address_____ Phone _____

Father's Name _____ Mother's Name _____

Brothers_____ Sisters _____ This child is _____ in family.
      Number   *Number*   *Number*

Has child ever attended a DISD school?   Yes _____ No _____ Where _____

1. How is health care provided for this student?   Employment Insurance ❏

    Private Insurance ❏   Social Security Insurance ❏   Medicaid ❏   Other ❏

2. With whom does child live?_____

3. When did your child have a physical examination? _____ _____
                                       Date   *Physician / Clinic*

    Purpose of examination: Routine check up ❏ Illness/Injury ❏ _____
                                                                       Specify

4. Does your child have a health problem? (Check where appropriate.)

    Asthma _____ Diabetes_____ Vision _____ Sickle Cell Anemia _____ Injury_____

    Allergies _____ Anemia _____ Hearing _____ Seizures/Convulsions _____ Heart_____

    Explain: _____

5. Does your child take medication? _____ Name of medication(s) _____
                                   Yes/No

6. During the pregnancy with this child, did the mother have any medical problems (e.g., high blood pressure or kidney infection, exposure to other infections)?_____

7. During the pregnancy with this child, did the mother smoke cigarettes? _____

    Amount _____

    Drink alcohol? _____ Amount _____

    Take any medication other than vitamins or iron?_____

    Name of medication(s) _____

Figure 2-2 (Continued)

8. Were there any problems during labor and delivery? _____

   Comments _____

   How long did the child remain in the hospital after birth? _____

   Did the child leave the hospital when his/her mother left? _____

   What age did your child: Walk alone? _____ Talk (2 words together)? _____

   Daytime toilet trained? _____

   Is bedwetting a problem? _____ If so, explain _____

9. Has child been hospitalized for any reason since birth? _____

10. Does any close relative in your family have a history of: (Check and indicate
    relationship to this child.)

    Diabetes _____   Cancer _____   High Blood Pressure _____

    Birth Defect _____   Anemia _____   Epilepsy _____

    Sickle Cell Anemia _____   Heart Disease _____   Learning Problems _____

    Mental Retardation _____   Other _____

11. Are there any problems in the home that might affect your child's learning? _____

    Comment: _____

12. Is there anything more about this child's health that you think is important for us

    to know? _____

Explain: _____

_____

_____   _____
                  Parent's Signature   *Date*

SCHOOL HEALTH SERVICE
HISTORIA CLINICA

Escuela _____

Grado _____

Estimados Padres:

Nos gustaría que su niño/a lograra el máximo de sus experiencias en la escuela. Para que nosotros podamos ayudarlo a lograr ésto, es necesario tener una historia clínica completa al corriente. Por favor, complete esta forma y regrésela al Director o a la enfermera de la escuela.

SU ENFERMERA ESCOLAR

Nombre del Alumno _____ _____ _____ Sexo _____ Fecha de nacimiento _____
(Apellido del padre) _(Nombre)_ _(Segundo Nombre)_

Dirección _____ Número de Teléfono _____

Nombre del Padre _____ Nombre de la Madre _____

Hermanos _____ Hermanas _____ Este niño/a es _____ en la familia.
(Número de) _(Número de)_ _(El Número)_

¿Alguna vez ha asistido su niño/a a una escuela del DISD? Sí _____ No _____ ¿Dónde? _____

1. ¿Qué seguro de salud tiene para su niño/a?   Seguro de su trabajo ☐
   Seguro Privado ☐   Seguro de Seguro Social ☐   Medicaid ☐   Otro ☐ _____

2. ¿Con quién vive el niño/a? _____

3. ¿Cuándo fué la última vez que su niño/a recibió un examen físico? _____ _____
   Fecha   _Médico/Clínica_

   Razón del examen: Examen de rutina ☐ Enfermedad/Herido ☐ _____
   Explique

4. ¿Tiene su niño/a un problema de salud? (Marcar donde es propio)
   Asma _____   Diabetes _____   Problemas de la vista _____   Drepanocito (sickle cell) _____   Herido _____
   Alergias _____   Anemia _____   Problemas del oído _____   Ataques/convulsiones _____
   Enfermedad del corazón _____   Otro: _____

   Explique: _____

5. ¿Toma su niño/a medicina(s)? _____ Nombre de medicina(s) _____
   _Si/No_

6. ¿Durante su embarazo con este/a niño/a, tuvo la madre problemas de salud _____
   (e.g., alta presión o infección del riñon, expuesta a otras infecciones)?

7. Durante su embarazo con este/a niño/a la madre fumó cigarillos? _____ Cantidad _____

   ¿Tomó bebidas alcohólicas? _____ Cantidad _____. Tomó medicina(s) aparte de vitaminas o hierro? _____

   Nombre de medicina(s) _____

8. ¿Tuvo problemas durante su parto? _____ Comentario _____

   ¿Cuánto tiempo duró su parto? _____ ¿Respiró el niño inmediatamente? _____ Peso al nacer _____

   ¿Cuánto tiempo duró el niño/a en el hospital después del nacimiento? _____

   ¿Se fué el niño/a a casa con su mamá? _____

   ¿A qué edad: Caminó solo su niño/a? _____ ¿Habló dos palabras juntas? _____ Empezó a usar el baño? _____

   ¿Moja la cama? _____ Si su repuesta es sí, por favor explicar. _____

9. ¿Ha sido su niño/a admitido en un hospital por alguna razón desde su nacimiento? _____

10. ¿Alguna persona en su familia tiene historia de: (Marque parentesco.)
    Diabetes _____   Cancer _____   Presión alta _____   Defecto de nacimiento _____
    Anemia _____   Epilepsia/Ataques _____   Drepanocito _____   Enfermedad del Corazón _____
    Problemas para aprender _____   Retardación Mental _____   Otro _____

11. ¿Hay problemas en su casa que podrán afectar el progreso para aprender de su niño/a? _____

    Commentario: _____

12. Nos puede decir algo de importancia de la salud de su niño/a que nosotros no le hayamos preguntado? _____

    Explique: _____

_____ Fecha _____
Firma del Padre

Figure 2-3

QUESTIONS FOR PHYSICIAN ABOUT A DISABLED STUDENT

1. What is the diagnosis?

2. What is the expected course of the condition? (static; progressive; fluctuating; fatal)

3. Does the child understand his/her condition?

4. Are there physical limitations or restrictions? (stairs, gym, excessive heat, etc.)

5. Is there a need to modify the student's schedule? (short day, homebound instruction, etc.)

6. Does the child take medication? Will it affect behavior? What are the side effects? Must it be given at school?

7. Does the child need special protective or other equipment?

8. Is a special procedure required during school hours? Are you willing to train the school nurse and/or other staff if necessary?

9. Should the child have preferential seating?

10. Is a modified diet needed at school?

11. Does the child need assistance with toileting?

12. Are there emotional or psychological issues to be considered?

13. Should the child receive special health counseling?

14. Are there emergency precautions to be taken by school staff? What hospital emergency room do you use?

15. Under what circumstance do you wish to be contacted?

16. Who is the alternate physician when you are not available?

17. Is there other information you wish to share with the school?

Figure 2-4

PHYSICIAN/PARENT REQUEST FOR ADMINISTRATION OF MEDICINE OR SPECIAL PROCEDURE BY SCHOOL PERSONNEL

Special health care procedures and medications may be administered at school by school personnel when such treatment is necessary for school attendance and cannot otherwise be accomplished. This completed form along with the medication and/or special equipment items are to be brought to the school by the parent.

Prescribed medication/treatment may be administered by a school nurse or by a non-health professional designate of the principal or school nurse. The medication should be brought to school in the original container appropriately labeled by the pharmacy. Parents may request that the pharmacist dispense two bottles of medication, one for home and one for school.

1. Name of Pupil _____ Birth Date _____

2. Address _____ School _____

3. Condition for which prescribed treatment is required:

4. Specific medication or procedure:

5. Dosage and method of administration/instruction (include time schedule):

6. Precautions, unfavorable reactions:

7. Disposition of pupil following administration or procedure, if applicable, i.e., rest, home, hospital, doctor's office, return to class.

8. Date of Request _____ Date of Termination _____

9. _____ / _____
   Physician's Name (printed)   *Signature*

   _____ / _____
   Physician's Address   *Telephone Number*

(PARENT)

We (I), the undersigned, the parents/guardians of _____
                                          Student's Name
request that the above medication or procedure be administered to our (my) child.

_____ / _____ Telephone _____ / _____
Name   *Relationship*   *Home*   *Business*

_____ / _____ Telephone _____ / _____
Name   *Relationship*   *Home*   *Business*

NOTE: Prescribed asthma inhaler may be kept by the student and self-administered if the physician indicates this need in writing and considers the student sufficiently responsible. In addition, the physician should list any precautions to be followed on this form (the school nurse will inform the principal and appropriate others).

SCHOOL HEALTH SERVICES

PARENT REQUEST FOR SPECIAL PROCEDURE BY SCHOOL PERSONNEL
PETICIÓN PATERNAL PARA PROCEDIMENTOS ESPECIALES DE SALUD EN LA ESCUELA

Special health care procedures may be performed by school personnel as follows/ *Procedimientos especiales para servicios de salud se pueden cumplir por medio del personal de la escuela como sigue:*
  1. When such treatment cannot otherwise be accomplished/*Cuando tal tratamiento no se puede cumplir de otra manera*
  2. On receipt of this completed form/*Al recibo de esta forma completada*

Mineral Oil may be administered at school by a non-health professional designate of the principal or school nurse/*El aceite mineral puede ser administrada en la escuela por medio de cualquier profesional designado por el director o la enfermera de la escuela.*

1. Name/*Nombre*_____ Age/*Edad*_____

2. Address/*Domicilio*_____ School/*Escuela*_____

3. Condition for which prescribed treatment is required/*Condición por la cual el tratamiento prescribido es requerido:*

   Ear canal(s) occluded with wax/*Canal(es) de oído(s) tapado(s) con cerilla.*

4. Specific procedure/*Procedimiento específico:*

   Mineral oil/warm water irrigation of canal(s)/*Aceite mineral/regamiento de canal(es) con agua tibia.*

5. Dosage and method of administration/*Dósis y método de administración:*
   Instruction for procedure/*Instrucciones del procedimiento:*
   Time(s)/*Hora(s)*_____

   Instill 2 drops of mineral oil twice daily for 3-5 days to Left/Right/Both ear(s). Procedure may be repeated if necessary./*Instilación de 2 gotas de aceite mineral dos veces al día de tres a cinco días, al oído izquierdo/derecho/los dos oídos. Quizá habrá necesidad de repetir el procedimiento.*

6. Precautions, unfavorable reactions/*Precauciones/reacciones adversas:*

	Yes/*Sí*	No
History of tubes in ears? *¿Hay historia médica de tubos en los oídos?*	—	—
Has your child complained of ear pain? *¿Se ha quejado de dolor en los oídos?*	—	—
Have you noticed any drainage from your child's ear(s)? *¿Ha notado algún derrame de los oídos?*	—	—

****

PARENT(S)/*PADRE(S):*

We (I), the undersigned, the parent(s)/guardian(s) of _____
Nosotros (Yo), infrascrito(s), padre(s)/curador(es) de Student/*Estudiante*

request the above procedure be administered to our (my) child.
pedimos que el procedimiento ya mencionado sea administrado a nuestro (mi) hijo/hija.

_____/_____Telephone_____/_____
Name/*Nombre* Relationship (*Teléfono*) Home/*Hogar* Business/*Negocio*
(*Parentesco*)

_____/_____Telephone_____/_____
Name/*Nombre* Relationship (*Teléfono*) Home/*Hogar* Business/*Negocio*
(*Parentesco*)

BY _____
FILED IN NURSE'S OFFICE ON _____

	Dates	Time	M	T	W	TH	F		Dates	Time	M	T	W	TH	F		Dates	Time	M	T	W	TH	F
1st								1st								1st							
2nd								2nd								2nd							

Figure 2-5

SCHOOL HEALTH SERVICES
INDIVIDUALIZED HEALTH PLAN (IHP)

NURSING DIAGNOSIS/ COLLABORATIVE PROBLEM	GOAL	PLAN OF ACTION	WHO
Intermittent impairment of oxygen exchange related to asthma	Student will demonstrate self-care procedures to become maximally independent.	Daily monitoring with peak flow meter (self-administered and recorded).	RN, health assistant, parent
		Monitor therapy ordered by M.D. Theophylline capsules Inhaled cromolyn sodium Inhaled albuteral as needed	RN, nurse aide
Impairment of physical activities related to suboptimum control of asthma.	Student will tolerate "normal" activities without fatigue or shortness of breath.	Review and monitor side effects of medication (nervousness,inattention, sweating, rash, hives).	Teacher, RN
		Encourage and monitor water intake.	RN, teacher, parent

Figure 2-6

HEALTH MANAGEMENT PLAN FOR
THE CHILD WITH ASTHMA

Asthma is a reversible obstructive lung disease with hyperreactive airways caused by a variety of stimuli. It is characterized by constriction of the bronchial smooth muscle, edema and inflammation of the mucous membranes lining the airways, and increased secretion of sticky mucous. The results are decreased air flow on inspiration and difficulty in expiring air from the lungs.

SIGNS OF AN ASTHMA ATTACK
1. coughing (often the earliest sign)
2. wheezing
3. rapid pulse (120 or greater)
4. labored breathing
5. increased use of accessory muscles of respiration

TRIGGERS OF ASTHMA (Varies from child to child)
1. environmental pollutants
2. exercise
3. cold air
4. emotions
5. infections

NOTE: The child who is having an asthma attack with significant respiratory distress is in even more danger when wheezing cannot be heard and breath sounds are minimal or absent.

NOTE: There is rarely only one triggering factor.

WHAT TO DO FOR AN ASTHMATIC CHILD

A. Prevention
1. Avoid known triggers if possible.
2. Promote exercise when child is asymtomatic. All activities should be endorsed by the child's physician.
3. Administer maintenance prescription medications.
4. Give child plenty of water, clear liquids, etc.

B. During an attack
1. Keep calm. Reassure the child by your tone of voice and your attitude that you are able to manage the situation.
2. Administer prescription medication for acute attack (if provided by parent/available).
3. Allow child to assume a position most comfortable for him/her and encourage relaxation.
4. Have student sip tap water slowly for hydration (not cold).
5. Instruct child to breathe in deeply, hold his/her breath 1 or 2 seconds, then cough twice—first to loosen mucous, and second to bring it up. Swallowed mucous may cause nausea and vomiting.

C. If condition does not improve
1. Notify parent and recommend immediate medical care. Send H16-Medical Referral Form.
2. In severe cases, summon emergency medical care services.

Figure 2-7

SPECIALIZED PROCEDURES IN THE SCHOOL SETTING

I. Medication Administration

    A. inhalation (nebulization)
    B. rectal
    C. bladder instillation
    D. gastric/NG tube
    E. intravenous
    F. IM, subcutaneous
    G. eye/nose drops

II. Feeding

    A. nasogastric / gastrostomy
    B. total parenteral (intravenous)

III. Catheterization (bladder)

    A. clean intermittent / sterile
    B. indwelling catheter care
    C. external catheter
    D. Credé maneuver

IV. Specimen Collecting and Testing

    A. blood glucose
    B. urine

V. Respiratory Procedures

    A. postural drainage / percussive therapy
    B. tracheostomy / oral suctioning
    C. continuous oxygen

VI. Intestinal Ostomies

    A. ostomy care
    B. ostomy irrigation

VII. Other Medical Support Systems

    A. ventriculoperitoneal shunts
    B. mechanical ventilator / respirator
    C. oxygen administration
    D. peritoneal dialysis
    E. apnea monitoring

Figure 2-8

SPECIAL EDUCATION DEPARTMENT—HOME/HOSPITAL BOUND PROGRAM—STATEMENT OF PHYSICIAN

Note to Physician:

Please check statement carefully and fill in *all* blanks in order to prevent delay in planning student's program. Return Originals and Duplicates.

_____/_____/_____/_____
   Student's Name, Last   *First*   *Middle*   *Birth Date*

_____ Home_____
       Student's Address   *Telephone*

For_____weeks the above-named student will be unable to attend a regular school or special class. [Physician must anticipate that the student will be absent for at least four (4) weeks.]

This student needs to continue school work at home or in the hospital under the Home/Hospital Bound Program, and this work will not interfere with recovery.

The student's illness (is) (is not) communicable, infectious, or contagious to others at this time.

Diagnosis of the student's illness is as follows:_____

_____

Are there other health problems?   ❏ YES   ❏ NO

If "YES," explain: _____

_____

Are there vision or hearing problems suspected?   ❏ YES   ❏ NO

If "YES," explain: _____

_____

Restrictions that the home/hospital teacher should observe in working with the student are as follows:

   1. Length of time for activity   _____

   2. Position: Flat _____. Upright _____. _____

   3. Length of sitting time _____

Precautions are as follows: _____

Prognosis for improvement is _____ *Prognosis* for life is _____

Return to:

_____
     Signature of Physician

_____
     Printed Name of Physician

_____
     Date

_____   _____
   Date Received   *Address of Physician*

Figure 2-9

SPECIAL EDUCATION DEPARTMENT
HOME/HOSPITAL BOUND PROGRAM

PHYSICIAN CLEARANCE TO RETURN TO SCHOOL

(Please return Original and Duplicates)

_____ / _____ / _____ / _____
Student's Name, Last   *First*   *Middle*   *Birth Date*

_____ Home _____ Business _____
     Student's Address   *Telephone*

The above-named student may return to school on _____

following an illness or incapacity of the following nature: _____

_____

_____

_____

_____

Limitations of activities are as follows: _____

_____

_____

_____

(Please state the length of time these limitations are to be observed): _____

_____

_____

_____

Other instructions regarding care of the student at school: _____

_____

_____

_____

This completed form should accompany the student upon returning to school from the Home/Hospital bound program.

_____
Signature of Physician

_____
Printed Name of Physician

_____
Date

_____
Address of Physician

_____
Office Telephone

CHAPTER 3

DEVELOPMENTAL AND EMOTIONAL PROBLEMS OF ELEMENTARY STUDENTS

Diagnosis of Mental Disorders
The Mind-Body Dilemma
School Readiness and Developmental Screening
Child Neglect or Abuse
Mental Retardation and Slow Learners
Learning Disabilities
Attention Deficit Hyperactivity Disorder (ADHD)
Psychosomatic Complaints
Conduct Disorder
Classroom Management Strategies
Other Developmental Disorders
Summary
References
Chapter 3 Figures:

Chapter 3

DEVELOPMENTAL AND EMOTIONAL PROBLEMS OF ELEMENTARY STUDENTS

It disappoints us to think that human beings . . . are not infinitely resilient.

Peter Kramer, 1993

This chapter and the next will deal with mental disorders first evident in childhood. The range is broad and extends from developmental delay and school readiness to psychosomatic complaints and conduct disorder. The intent is to set out broad categories of emotional and developmental problems that are similar in their management requirements. Early recognition and referral by you are of prime importance.

DIAGNOSIS OF MENTAL DISORDERS

To adequately understand and deal with these problems, you should have a working knowledge of the classifications contained in the *Diagnostic and Statistical Manual of Mental Disorders* (American Psychiatric Association, 1994). The *DSM*, as it is called, is the gold standard for diagnosis used by psychiatrists, psychologists, and other mental health professionals. Criteria are given for the diagnosis of each condition. The use of the *DSM* as a standard allows greater precision and uniformity of terminology, and improves communication among professionals and from professionals to parents and children. The following is an abbreviated table of contents:

- Mental Retardation
- Learning Disorders (dyslexia, dyscalculia)

- Motor Skills Disorder (developmental coordination disorder)
- Pervasive Developmental Disorders (autistic disorder)
- Disruptive Behavior and Attention Deficit Disorders (conduct disorder, ADHD)
- Eating Disorders (pica, anorexia, bulimia)
- Tic Disorders (Tourette's, etc.)
- Communication Disorders (expressive / receptive language disorders)
- Elimination Disorders (encopresis, enuresis)
- Other Disorders of Infancy, Childhood, or Adolescence (separation anxiety, elective mutism, habit disorder)

An important fact to keep in mind is that these general categories are not mutually exclusive. For example, a child can have ADHD plus conduct disorder, or mental retardation and stereotyped movement.

THE MIND-BODY DILEMMA

In Chapter 2, epilepsy was used as an example of a condition in which it is often difficult to separate body from mind. When cognitive impairment is present, how much is related to the underlying epilepsy? In a British study published in 1993 (*Developmental Medicine and Child Neurology*, Vol. 35, pp. 574–81), the authors report a trial of anti-epileptic medication to treat cognitive defects due to subclinical epileptiform EEG discharges in children with psychosocial and educational problems associated with epilepsy. In all instances, epileptiform activity (assessed by 24 hour, ambulatory EEG monitoring) was reduced compared with that of a placebo group. In general, there was improvement of psychosocial function. These findings support the view that subclinical EEG discharges can impair psychosocial function and may respond to anti-epileptic medication.

Despite the incompleteness of our knowledge (psychiatry is still an inexact science), it is useful to attempt to separate primary from secondary emotional problems. The usefulness comes in developing management strategies and specific treatments. In the above report, the cognitive problems were primary (related to the epilepsy) and not secondary (psychogenic). To complicate matters further, the same child with epilepsy and primary cognitive or behavioral problems may (and often does) have secondary emotional problems related to low self-esteem because of the physical and social limitations imposed by the chronic condition.

The point is that rarely are you dealing with students who have purely physical or purely emotional problems. Mind and body each know what the other is doing and usually signal us in ways we can recognize. With this knowledge, the professional and the affected individual can better manage a given set of problems. The pronouncement, "it's all in her head" has become a historical footnote—more under psychosomatic complaints.

SCHOOL READINESS AND DEVELOPMENTAL SCREENING

Sometimes you will be asked to help decide if a child is ready for school. More often, you will be asked to participate in the evaluation of a student who is already enrolled—one who seems "immature" for his age—it *is* more often a male.

I will dispense with the concept of delayed enrollment first. It is rare that the needs of the "unready" child will be met by simply keeping the child at home. While developmental skills do improve with time alone, they improve much more rapidly in a stimulating educational setting. When I encounter parents (usually high achieving) who want to delay school enrollment so their child "will be competitive," I try to dissuade them. Failing that, I strongly encourage a good preschool setting. At this stage of decision making, developmental testing is not terribly helpful except for identifying mental retardation. No test to date has succeeded in predicting academic skills before those skills are supposed to be present developmentally; that is, our success at forecasting reading ability in four-year-olds is poor (Black, 1990).

A related concept is repeating a grade. Although frequently recommended, repeating a grade does not help a student gain ground academically and has a negative impact on social adjustment and self-esteem.

It *is* helpful to know how a child compares with peers in terms of motor skills, language, attention, and social-emotional status. This starting point is essential to planning an appropriate program for a given child. It has been my experience that kindergarten and first grade teachers fare as well as formal assessments in spotting students who will need extra help.

The characteristics of a developmentally appropriate kindergarten classroom are as follows.

- Different ability levels and learning styles are expected.
- Children select many of their own activities.
- Children are expected to be physically and mentally active.
- Opportunities are provided to see how reading and writing are useful before children are instructed in letter names.
- Learning about math is integrated into meaningful activities such as measuring water in food preparation.
- Group size is limited to 10 to 15 students per adult.

CHILD NEGLECT OR ABUSE

School personnel have, for the most part, done a good job of recognizing the signs of physical abuse. They are generally less adept at recognizing the early signs of subtle neglect, or emotional and sexual abuse. The topic is too broad for this work, but suffice it to say that any inappropriate or strange behavior in a child should be investigated with the potential for abuse in mind. Two examples of such behaviors are seeking affection from strangers (ages five and above) and severe social withdrawal. Both extremes can have their roots in abusive or neglectful caretakers.

MENTAL RETARDATION AND SLOW LEARNERS

Although the literature on this subject is extensive, one concept bears mentioning: mental age. While the pitfalls of IQ testing are significant, knowing the approximate mental age of a child is helpful. Figure 3-1, at the end of this chapter, gives the mental ages for children from 5 through 11 years for IQs between 55 and 80.

These figures can be calculated for any age and IQ by using the formula for the ratio IQ:

$$IQ = \frac{Mental\ age\ (months)}{Chronological\ age\ (months)} \times 100$$

Solving for mental age we get

$$MA = \frac{IQ \times CA}{100}$$

Thus, knowing the IQ and chronological age, you can determine the approximate mental age. Use months for both MA and CA, then divide your answer by 12 to get MA in years.

Armed with the mental age of a child (which correlates reasonably well with receptive language age) you can pitch your questions and instructions at an appropriate level. For instance, if you are trying to explain menstrual care to a 12-year-old with an IQ of 55, it is clear you must do so in terms that a $6\frac{1}{2}$-year-old would understand.

Children whose IQs fall between 70 and 89 are described as slow learners. Of course, these numbers are somewhat arbitrary as the progression from mental retardation, through slow learner, to normal intelligence is a smooth continuum. Students who are slow learners often fall through the cracks because they don't usually qualify for special education, yet they have difficulty in the regular classroom. This group is at great risk for emotional problems secondary to multiple academic failures. Figure 3-2 illustrates the IQ range for slow learners and other developmental disabilities.

LEARNING DISABILITIES

Dyslexia is perhaps the best known of the specific developmental learning disabilities. The term *dyslexia* refers to a student who is more than a year behind in reading level despite adequate educational opportunities. Conditions that could cause the reading delay have also been ruled out (mental retardation, vision and hearing loss, primary emotional disorder, inadequate teaching, etc.). A more current term for these students is specific reading disability.

Poor reading ability is the cause of more academic underachievement than any other cause. Unfortunately, remedial reading instruction is laborious and produces slow progress. It also robs time from other subjects and may reduce self-esteem. Informed educators are now recommending that remedial reading not be too intensive or carried on for too long. Acquisition of information and concepts is the key element in education. If reading disability has slowed the flow of information (inability to complete reading assignments), bypass techniques should be used—any method that bypasses the printed word and allows for continued information input to the child. Examples include tape recordings (audiocassettes, videotapes), laser discs, and computers. Allowing LD students to take untimed tests is another accommodation. It is inexcusable for a child with a normal IQ to have his or her information flow slowed by a reading disability. The problem is compounded as reading assignments increase in the upper elementary grades.

Many dyslexic adults do not progress beyond a fifth- or sixth-grade reading level and continue to be poor spellers. They generally have minimal expressive language problems. For these individuals, the earlier we begin to bypass the print barrier, the brighter their future will be. You can serve as an important advocate for these future citizens.

ATTENTION DEFICIT HYPERACTIVITY DISORDER (ADHD)

Much has been written on this subject, yet our understanding of it remains incomplete. Nevertheless, we must try to help these students gain maximum benefit from their educational opportunity. The main stumbling block is inattention. They are distractible and can't concentrate on an activity as long as their peers. Despite normal or above normal intelligence, they usually do not fare well when report card time arrives.

The hyperactivity part of this disorder is present in varying degrees and contributes to the challenge of sitting still and paying attention. Those children with minimal hyperactivity are the last to be recognized and diagnosed because their inattention may go unnoticed by the teacher if they are not disruptive to the class.

The most severely affected children are easily recognized by the classroom teacher, but they may be able to control their behavior during short-term formal assessments (psychological testing; visits to the doctor's office). Teacher check-lists are essential in documenting variant behaviors for other professionals. One user-friendly screening tool is the Conners' Abbreviated Teacher's School Report. See Figure 3-3.

The total possible score for the ten items is 30 (most severely affected child). The average cutoff score for an ADHD child is 15. Figure 3-4 demonstrates specific cutoff scores by gender and ethnicity. It is apparent that a score of 15 would warrant an ADHD referral for all Hispanics and white females, but not for white males or Blacks. The minimum score for a referral of a Black male is 19 (out of 30). These cutoff scores will not identify attention deficit in the absence of hyperactivity. Items 4 and 6 (relating to attention span) must be considered in isolation for these children; if they are both 3s, attention deficit is likely.

Although the Conners' abbreviated scale is merely a screening (*not* diagnostic) instrument, it is an important first step in an objective evaluation process. Many similar instruments are available and useful.

Once a child is identified as possibly ADHD by the teacher checklist, a referral should be made to a physician for consideration of a medication such as methylphenidate (Ritalin). While it is not a magic bullet, many ADHD children are markedly improved on this prescription drug.

Simultaneously, the potential ADHD student who is underachieving should receive formal psychoeducational testing. Approximately half of ADHD students will have a coexisting learning disability (such as dyslexia). This testing may be done within the school system or by an outside professional.

Whether a child receives or benefits from medication or not, classroom management is paramount. Psychologists are generally the best people to make these recommendations to classroom teachers and parents. Recommendations should be in writing (part of a child's IEP) and understood and practiced by all adults who interact with the child (see the section on classroom management strategies in this chapter). If medication is prescribed, the teacher checklist can be used again in two to three weeks to see if improvement can be documented. Ritalin or other drugs, when helpful, are usually continued until puberty. At that time, a decision is made to discontinue or continue the treatment. If attention span is still improved, it should be continued.

Stimulant drugs used by ADHD children do not produce addiction, but should be controlled by an adult.

PSYCHOSOMATIC COMPLAINTS

The concept of psychosomatic pain is one that is invoked entirely too often. It has become the wastebasket when we can't find a cause for the problem. You may be tempted to use this label with frequent clinic visitors. If it is to be a valid diagnostic label, the pain (or other complaint) must not only be manifested in the absence of identifiable organic (physical) disease but be accompanied by positive personality characteristics that mental health professionals categorize as neuroses.

The term *psychogenesis* implies an origin of symptoms (such as headache or stomachache) in the mind, usually due to obvious stress or to troubling thoughts in the subconscious (remembering negative experiences or "abnormal desires"). The inference is, if I am in pain, it is because my unconscious (or subconscious) mind is thinking pain. My conscious mind responds by perceiving pain somewhere in the body: stomach pain even though the stomach is perfectly well, headaches even though I do not have migraine or a brain tumor.

The most common psychosomatic scenario I have encountered in the school setting is the high-achieving 9–10-year-old female with stomachache. It is a challenge to manage because you don't want to discourage striving for good grades. Neither is an automatic psychiatric referral a good idea; it plants the seed of "mental disorder" in the mind of the child, parents, and teachers. What to do? An experienced counselor, psychologist, or nurse can often, through an in-depth interview, identify significant concerns and stressors in the child's conscious mind. Others (subconscious) may be inferred by knowing the child's total environment and behaviors in specific situations. Recommendations often fall under the rubric of reducing parental and self-imposed pressure to perform.

I try to put things in perspective for parents and child (and sometimes teachers) by stating that most colleges prefer B students who have extracurricular activities to straight A students with none. I am always amazed at how often this simple piece of information is accepted and acted on. Get a hobby—get a life!

We must be humble, patient and persistent when we can't find a reason for a child's symptoms.

CONDUCT DISORDER

The *DSM* (*Diagnostic and Statistical Manual of Mental Disorders,* 4th edition) defines conduct disorder as a persistent violation of the basic rights of others or of major age-appropriate norms of society. Physical aggression is common. Examples include cruelty to animals, property destruction, fire setting, lying, and covert stealing. The behavior pattern typically is present in the home, at school, with peers, and in the community. While the diagnosis of conduct disorders is the purview of mental health professionals, primary providers should be able to recognize the early signs and make a referral.

The specific diagnostic criteria for conduct disorder include a disturbance of conduct lasting at least six months, during which at least three of the following are present:

- has stolen without confrontation of a victim on more than one occasion
- has run away from home overnight at least twice

- often lies
- deliberately engaged in fire-setting
- is often truant from school
- has broken into someone else's house, building, or car
- has deliberately destroyed others' property
- has been physically cruel to animals
- has forced someone into sexual activity
- has used a weapon in more than one fight
- often initiates physical fights
- has stolen with confrontation of a victim
- has been physically cruel to people

Conduct disorder often persists into adulthood and is then termed antisocial personality disorder. It is often preceded by oppositional defiant disorder—a milder form seen in younger children. Many of the affected children also have ADHD and specific learning disabilities. Figure 3-5 illustrates the progression sometimes seen without proper and early intervention.

The diagnostic criteria for oppositional defiant disorder include a disturbance of at least six months during which at least five of the following are present:

- often loses temper
- often argues with adults
- often actively defies or refuses adult requests or rules
- often deliberately does things that annoy other people
- often blames others for his or her own mistakes
- is often touchy or easily annoyed by others
- is often angry and resentful
- is often spiteful or vindictive
- often swears or uses obscene language.

CLASSROOM MANAGEMENT STRATEGIES

The following suggestions are adapted from Cardwell* (1990, unpublished) and apply primarily for ADHD students but are, for the most part, applicable to oppositional defiant disorder and other behavioral disorders:

---

*From Milton Cardwell, M.D., F.A.A.P., Private Practice of Developmental and Behavioral Pediatrics, Irving, Texas.

- Arrange preferential seating close to the teacher (away from hall noise, pencil sharpeners, and other distractions).
- Nurture positive self-esteem (never intentionally humiliate).
- Maintain confidentiality from peers regarding diagnosis and medication (never say, "Did you take your pill?" out loud in class).
- Keep a highly structured classroom with a set schedule.
- Divide work load into small units.
- Alternate difficult and easy tasks.
- Give frequent positive reinforcement for successes.
- Consider use of a study carrel for individual assignments.
- Provide opportunities to express motoric restlessness (prearranged errands).
- Limit instructions to two steps at a time (pause and let these be carried out before giving a third and fourth step).
- Be the child's advocate (discourage outside value judgments by classmates).
- Keep a sense of humor and comradeship about the many challenges the student presents.

The classroom teacher can make a difference in how this student perceives himself or herself and others. This in turn will make a difference in how he or she performs.

OTHER DEVELOPMENTAL DISORDERS

Three additional disorders are worth a brief mention:
- Pervasive Developmental Disorder
- Tic disorders
- Motor skills disorder

Pervasive Developmental Disorder (PDD)

Formerly called childhood schizophrenia, this disorder is devastatingly severe and has a poor prognosis. It has many of the features of mental retardation, but the affected child is less socialized; some are entirely introverted and fail to interact with their environment. Autism is a subset of this condition, but its relation to adult psychosis is unclear. Only a small minority of these individuals are able to lead independent lives; most remain severely disabled, with marked signs of the disorder. Factors related to long-term outcomes include IQ and the development of social and language skills.

Tic Disorders

A tic is an involuntary, sudden, rapid, recurrent, nonrhythmic, stereotyped (always the same) motor movement or vocalization. Tics are often made worse by stress and usually are markedly diminished during sleep. They may also lessen during absorbing activities such as reading. Tourette's Syndrome is the severest form of tic disorder. The essential features of this disorder are multiple motor and one or more vocal tics. Facial grimaces are the most common motor tics seen. Vocal tics include throat clearing or coughing, barking, grunting, and sniffing. Coprolalia (uttering obscenities) is seen in approximately half the cases. The first symptoms to appear are bouts of a single tic, most frequently eye blinking. If manifestations are less than the full-blown Tourette's Syndrome, it may be termed *transient tic disorder,* or *chronic motor* or *vocal tic disorder.*

The major tranquilizer haloperidol (Haldol) is often used to treat Tourette's. Stimulants such as methylphenidate (Ritalin) make tics worse and are contraindicated.

Motor Skills Disorder

Developmental Coordination Disorder is the official *DSM* name for this condition. It is sometimes referred to as the "clumsy child syndrome." The essential feature is a marked impairment in the development of motor coordination that is not explained by mental retardation and that is not due to a known physical disorder. This diagnosis is made by mental health professionals only if the impairment significantly interferes with academics (poor handwriting, etc.) or with activities of daily living. Young children have difficulty tying shoelaces, buttoning, and zipping. Older students display difficulty with puzzle assembly, model building, playing ball, and handwriting. The prevalence is estimated to be as high as 6% for children in the age range 5–11 years. The course is variable, but in some cases, lack of coordination continues through adolescence to adulthood.

SUMMARY

The *DSM* is the standard for the diagnosis of mental disorders used by psychiatrists and psychologists. You should have a working knowledge of the categories it contains, remembering that diagnostic categories often overlap and many are not mutually exclusive.

Beyond these diagnostic categories each child must be assessed *functionally* in terms of general physical health, motor and cognitive skills, social skills, academic skills, and environmental background (home and school). Only then can we begin with the child where he or she is, and build on strengths and repair or bypass deficits. Rigid diagnostic categories and cook-book approaches to management should be taken *cum grano salis*. Strive for a holistic approach within the boundaries of your expertise. A good working relationship with school psychologists and counselors is essential to optimum management of children with behavioral and emotional problems.

REFERENCES

1. Bagnato, S. *Linking Developmental Assessment and Curricula.* Rockville, MD: Aspen, 1981.

2. Berman, S. In "Behavioral and Developmental Disorders" *Pediatric Decision Making.* Philadelphia: B. C. Decker, Inc., 1991, pp. 358–403.

3. Black, J. "School Readiness." *Pediatric Basics,* Gerber Medical Service, no. 55 (Summer 1990), pp. 2–5.

4. —. *Diagnostic and Statistical Manual of Mental Disorders (DSM,* 3d edition, revised). Washington, DC: American Psychiatric Association, 1987.

5. —. *DSM-IV Draft Criteria.* Washington, DC: American Psychiatric Association, 1993.

6. Frankenburg, W. "Preventing Developmental Delays." *Pediatrics* 93(4):586–593.

7. Herskowitz, J. *Pediatrics, Neurology and Psychiatry—Common Ground.* New York: Macmillan, 1982.

8. Hill, Austin. *Why Students Fail.* Waco, Texas: Davis Brothers Publishing, 1991.

9. Keele, D. *The Developmentally Disabled Child.* Oradell, NJ: Medical Economics Books, 1983.

10. Lewis, R. "Coordinating Services for the Young Developmentally Disabled Patient." *Physician Assistant* (October 1992): 68–73.

11. McDonald, P. "Are You Missing Developmental Disabilities?" *Physician Assistant* (August 1992): 31–34.

12. Millon, T. (ed). *Contemporary Directions in Psychopathology.* New York: The Guilford Press, 1986.

13. Nader, P. R. (ed). "Behavior Discipline Problems" in *School Health: Policy and Practice,* pp. 177–187. Elk Grove Village, IL: American Academy of Pediatrics, 1993.

14. —. "The Pediatrician and the New Morbidity." *Pediatrics* 92(5):731–733.

15. Shorter, E. *From the Mind into the Body: The Cultural Origins of Psychosomatic Symptoms.* New York: Free Press (Macmillan), 1994.

Figure 3-1

APPROXIMATE MENTAL AGE OF
RETARDED STUDENTS*

IQ Age	55	60	65	70	75	80
5 (60 mo.)	2.8	3.0	3.3	3.5	3.8	4.0
6 (72 mo.)	3.3	3.6	4.0	4.2	4.5	4.8
7 (84 mo)	3.9	4.2	4.6	4.9	5.3	5.6
8 (96 mo.)	4.4	4.8	5.2	5.6	6.0	6.4
9 (108 mo.)	5.0	5.4	5.9	6.0	6.8	7.2
10 (120 mo.)	5.5	6.0	6.5	7.0	7.5	8.0
11 (132 mo.)	6.0	6.5	7.1	7.7	8.2	8.8
12 (144 mo.)	6.5	7.1	7.8	8.4	9.0	9.5

* Based on simple ratio IQ.

Figure 3-2

IQ DISTRIBUTION IN THE VARIOUS DEVELOPMENTAL DISABILITIES

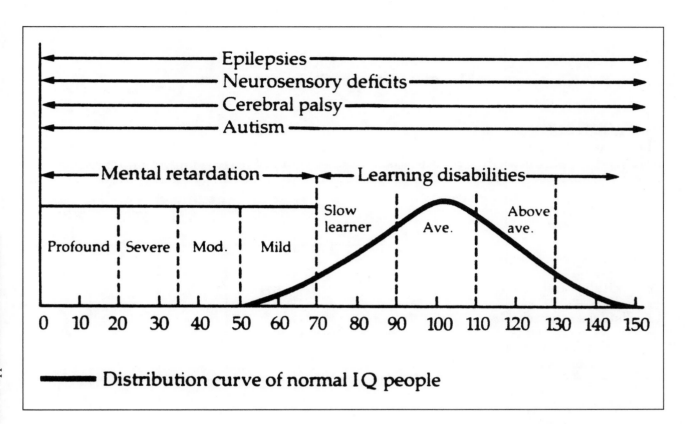

Figure 3-3

Name _____ School _____

Date _____ Age _____ Grade_____ Birth Date _____

Time of Day _____ a.m.
p.m.   Subject _____

CONNERS'
Abbreviated Teacher's School Report

INSTRUCTIONS:

Check the appropriate box for each item, **Not at all, Just a little, Pretty much,** or **Very much,** which best describes your assessment of the child. Please complete all ten items.

Observation	Degree of Activity			
	0 Not at all	**1** Just a little	**2** Pretty much	**3** Very much
1. Restless or overactive				
2. Excitable, impulsive				
3. Disturbs other children				
4. Fails to finish things he/she starts, short attention span				
5. Constantly fidgeting				
6. Inattentive, easily distracted (interferes with learning)				
7. Demands must be met immediately—easily frustrated				
8. Cries often and easily				
9. Mood changes quickly and drastically				
10. Temper outbursts, explosive and unpredictable behavior				

Initiated by _____   _____
                    Health Professional   *Observer's Signature*

                                        Disposition _____
                                                            Health Professional

COMMENTS:

Figure 3-4

CUTOFF SCORES ON THE CONNERS' SCALE
BY ETHNICITY AND GENDER*

SEX	BLACK	WHITE	HISPANIC
Male	19	16	13
Female	16	14	12

*Age is not a significant variable between six and nine years. Scores indicate the top 10% in each gender/ethnic subgroup (minimum score for ADHD referral).

Figure 3-5

PROGRESSION OF SYNDROMES

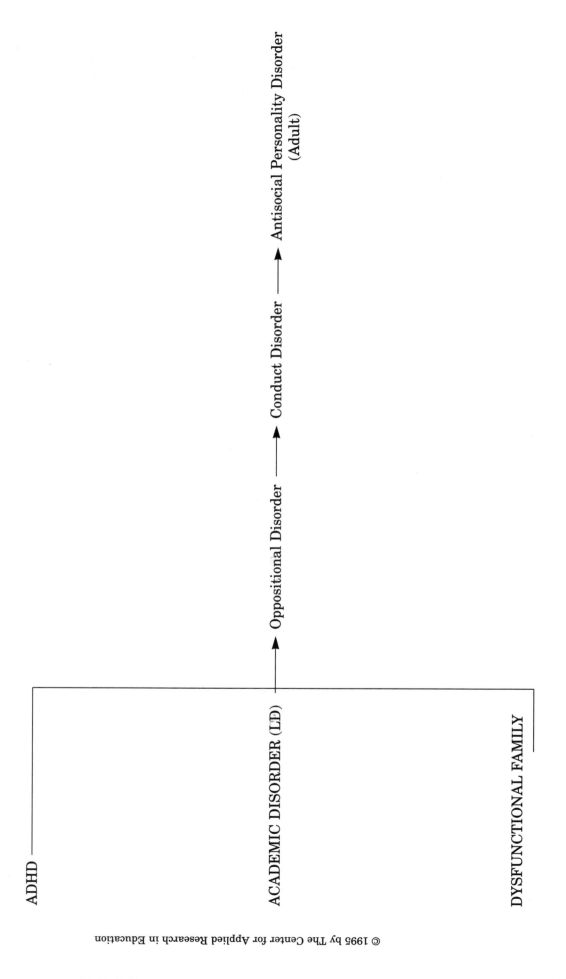

ADHD

ACADEMIC DISORDER (LD) ⟶ Oppositional Disorder ⟶ Conduct Disorder ⟶ Antisocial Personality Disorder (Adult)

DYSFUNCTIONAL FAMILY

CHAPTER 4

BEHAVIORAL AND EMOTIONAL PROBLEMS OF ADOLESCENTS

Chapter 4

BEHAVIORAL AND EMOTIONAL PROBLEMS OF ADOLESCENTS

At thirteen we have so many choices to make, with no idea how consequences can rattle through the decades.

Michael Cunningham, 1990

For most students, the teen years are a time for physical and mental development, not of illness. When illness occurs, it is often related to the increased risk-taking behavior that is part of normal adolescent exploration. Unfortunately, exploration can be dangerous.

The major cause of mortality in adolescents nationally is motor vehicle accidents; more than half are related to drug or alcohol use. Next in importance are homicide and suicide.

Causes of morbidity in adolescents include drug abuse, sexually transmitted diseases (STD), eating disorders, and symptoms related to stress and depression. None of these are easily amenable to intervention; in fact, new morbidity disorders may not even show up in the standard health history and review of systems (ROS) we are taught to perform.

When you see adolescents, you must be willing to take an adequate psychosocial history. If this is not done, there is little chance of spotting problems early and making a significant impact on morbidity and mortality.

Obtaining an accurate psychosocial history depends on trust. Teenage students must feel that the school nurse

- is interested in them.
- can help with solutions to problems.
- will maintain confidentiality.

It is unreasonable to expect a young person to reveal personal information unless confidentiality can be assured. It should be explained to students that confidences will be kept unless an individual is in danger or poses a serious threat to others. Driving while intoxicated, expressing suicidal wishes, and admitting sexual abuse are situations in which a confidence should *not* be kept. With the exceptions noted, it should be a goal to have the student reveal sensitive information to parents or other authority figures.

GETTING INSIDE THE ADOLESCENT'S HEAD

A useful checklist for the psychosocial interview has been published by Goldenring (*Contemporary Pediatrics*, July 1988). The acronym HEADSS guides the interviewer through the process.

H—home
E—education / employment
A—activities
D—drugs
S—sexuality
S—suicide / depression

Key questions for each of the six areas should be answered by the teen *and* a parent.

Home: Who lives there? Whom can the teen talk to? What do parents or guardians do for a living? What are relationships like? Any family member ever incarcerated or institutionalized? Recent moves? Running away? New people in home environment?

Education/Employment: School performance? Recent changes? Favorite subjects? Worst subjects? Any years repeated? Current job? Change of schools? Future plans?

Activities: What do you do for fun? With peers? With family? Clubs? Sports or exercise? Church? Hobbies? TV? Reading? Music? Drive a car? History of acting out or arrests?

Drugs: Use by peers? Use by teen (include alcohol and tobacco)? Use by family members?

Sexuality: Orientation? Types of sexual experience? Number of partners? Masturbation? (normalize), History of pregnancy? Sexually transmitted diseases? Contraception? History of abuse?

Suicide / Depression: Long-lasting blue moods? Appetite change? Trouble sleeping? Boredom? Thoughts of death? Ever considered taking his or her life? Seen a mental health professional? Therapy?

The HEADSS interview is brief enough to be administered to all teens seen for comprehensive health care or a specific behavioral problem. It should be administered only after trust has been developed—sometimes on a second visit. Make it clear that these questions are asked of *all* adolescents you see. Acknowledge that they are very personal and answers will remain confidential. It is also helpful to note the student's body language during responses.

If the young person cannot trust or talk to anyone at home, you can prepare the way for trust in other significant adults.

ANXIETY DISORDERS

Anxiety is a feeling of dread and apprehension about the future. It has also been referred to as chronic fear. Anxiety is a subjective symptom that cannot be quantified easily but there are usually physical manifestations (not all will be present in the same student).

- restlessness
- muscle tension or trembling
- tachycardia
- rapid breathing
- sweating
- flushing

Anxiety is a part of life when dealing with challenging situations. It can be considered normal unless it results in significant avoidance behavior. Deciding what constitutes normal versus pathological anxiety can be difficult. An adolescent must tell you how distressed he or she feels—the subjective experience is important. Try to judge whether the anxiety is appropriate to the situation.

Be aware that individuals may not complain of anxiety as such (especially younger teens). Complaints of lightheadedness, tingling extremities, hyperventilation, and sense of "unreality" are often expressions of anxiety.

Primary Anxiety Disorders

Primary anxiety conditions include phobias, panic attacks, generalized anxiety, post-traumatic stress disorders, obsessive-compulsive disorders, and dissociative episodes. A few are briefly described.

Phobias—Illogical fears of situations, animals, places, etc. They are single or isolated (only one phobia per customer) and are appreciated by the individual as being illogical.

Desensitization Therapy—gradually increasing the exposure of the patient to the feared situation—usually lessens phobias. Some common phobias are fear of heights (acrophobia), fear of spiders (arachnophobia) and fear of open spaces (agoraphobia).

Panic Attacks—Discrete periods of intense fear or discomfort accompanied by one or more of the physical manifestations listed earlier. In addition, some of the following subjective symptoms are also present: shortness of breath, dizziness, palpitations, choking, nausea, tingling of the fingers, chest pain, feeling of unreality, and fear of dying or going crazy. Unexpected onset is an essential feature. Medical conditions (hyperthyroidism) and drug toxicity (amphetamines) must be ruled out.

Obsessive-Compulsive Disorder—A psychoneurosis characterized by persistent and often unwanted ideas (obsessions) and impulses to carry out irrational, stereotyped and ritualistic acts (compulsions). Obsessive-compulsive behaviors are considered attempts to overcome anxiety or to lessen guilt feelings. For example, the handwashing compulsion may reflect the individual's anxiety and guilt about masturbation.

School Phobia—This term is a misnomer as it does not represent a fear of school per se. Rather it is a separation anxiety centering around an important caretaker, usually the mother. The essential feature is persistent worry about possible harm befalling the mother, or that she will leave and not return. Affected children may have physical complaints: headache, stomachache, nausea, or vomiting.

Boys, especially, may deny concern about their mother or their wish to be with her, yet their behavior reflects anxiety about separation. This disorder, in the broadest sense, represents a form of phobia, but always has its onset before the age of 18. Depressed mood is frequently present.

It should be noted that a small number of school refusal cases are not due to separation anxiety. Here, the adolescents actually fear the school situation because of anxiety about social or academic performance.

Individuals with separation anxiety are often demanding, intense, and in need of constant attention. They may complain that no one loves them and they wish they were dead, especially if separation is enforced. Others are described as unusually conscientious, compliant, and eager to please. When the need for separation is dealt with sensitively, individuals with separation anxiety disorder have no interpersonal difficulties; they tend to come from families that are close-knit.

Onset of the disorder in adolescence is rare, but persistence from childhood to adolescence is not. It may even extend to resistance to going away to college.

Avoidant Disorder

The essential feature of this disorder is an excessive shrinking from contact with unfamiliar people. It is severe enough to interfere with social functioning in peer relationships, and is coupled with a clear preference for social involvement with familiar people. Relationships with family members and other familiar figures are warm and satisfying.

When the youngster enters school, the manifestations imitate separation anxiety (school phobia), but in this case there is an actual fear of strangers. Females are affected more often than males, and the disorder may continue into adulthood.

Overanxious Disorder

The criteria for this disorder are

- excessive or unrealistic worry about future events
- excessive or unrealistic worry about the appropriateness of past behavior
- concern about competence in one or more areas (academic, athletic, social)
- somatic complaints (stomachache, headache)
- marked self-consciousness
- excessive need for reassurance
- inability to relax

This disorder interferes with meeting demands at school. The affected young person has often had multiple medical evaluations for the somatic complaints. It is more common in hyperachieving families in the upper socioeconomic bracket. Males and females are equally affected.

Perspective on Anxiety

It should be clear that various types of anxiety disorders have certain features in common and some may co-exist in the same person. Most of the manifestations are subjective and criteria for diagnosis are imprecise at best. In fact, two psychiatrists may diagnose the same individual differently (this is not unknown in the realm of physical ailments either).

Your most important role is to refer students with chronic manifestations of anxiety to the school psychologist or an outside mental health professional. Falling grades, increased time in the school clinic, or increased absences are red flags for referral. If the child has already been diagnosed and is on medication, your role is to report progress and regressions.

EATING DISORDERS

This group of conditions is characterized by gross disturbances in eating behavior. There are two related conditions in this category: anorexia nervosa and bulimia. The usual onset is in adolescence.

Anorexia nervosa (AN)

"Anorexia" is a misnomer since loss of appetite is rare. The essential features of anorexia nervosa are

- refusal to maintain body weight above minimum normal for age and height
- intense fear of becoming fat
- distorted body image (thinking one looks fat even when thin)
- amenorrhea
- reduction in food intake (often with extensive exercising)

Affected individuals generally come to medical attention when they reach 85% of ideal weight. They may even be suspected of having a malignancy. Physical signs often include hypothermia, low blood pressure, slow heart rate, edema, and cessation of menstrual periods. Students with AN deny the severity of the illness and may resist treatment.

Many of these adolescents have delayed sexual development and a diminished interest in sex. Females represent 95% of the cases. In 5% the course is unremitting until death; however, the more common course (with proper management) is a return to normal weight.

Bulimia

Bulimia is characterized by binge eating followed by self-induced catharsis (vomiting or use of laxatives or diuretics). Unlike AN, weight does not fall below minimum levels for age and height.

Other essential features include

- feeling of lack of control over eating
- periods of strict dieting
- vigorous exercise
- overconcern with body shape and weight
- fluctuating weight

Binge eating is done in secret and includes large amounts of high-calorie sweets. Binges are terminated by abdominal discomfort. Although eating binges may be pleasurable, self-criticism and depressed mood often follow. Affected individuals feel that their lives are dominated by conflicts about eating. Some are subject to substance abuse, particularly amphetamines for their anticipated appetite suppressant effects. Alcohol abuse is also seen. Certain activity groups and professions are at greater risk: dancers, gymnasts, track participants, swimmers, models, and aspiring actors.

Onset is usually in adolescence or early adulthood and the course is chronic and intermittent over many years. Complications include erosion of tooth enamel (from hydrochloric acid in vomitus), dehydration, electrolyte imbalance, and tears of the stomach or esophagus from retching. Females are much more often affected than males, and most of these are white and upper middle class. Bulimia is not as often fatal as AN but it can interfere significantly with school, both academically and socially. It has been called the prototype of psychosomatic disorders, but there are no totally satisfactory theories to explain its cause. The distinction between bulimia and AN is confusing as the two may overlap or occur in the same adolescent at different times.

School nurses should remember that not all students who try to lose weight develop an eating disorder. Neither will the school nurse induce AN or bulimia by recommending weight loss. Simple obesity is a much greater problem in the school-age population.

Concomitant depression occurs in about 50% of individuals with AN and suicide is the most common cause of death. About one-third of bulimics have conduct problems that may include stealing food, sexual promiscuity, and drug or alcohol abuse.

Treatment of Bulimia and Anorexia Nervosa

Anorexia and bulimia both have significant medical and psychological consequences. Hospitalization is often indicated to correct medical problems quickly (malnutrition, electrolyte imbalance, etc.), and initiate psychiatric evaluation. Individual or group psychotherapy provides the cornerstone of effective treatment. Medications are sometimes used to diminish anxiety. Drug treatment of associated depression is also indicated.

Prevention efforts (focusing on educating young adolescents and their families about the risks of dieting and unrealistic role models thrust on women) are needed to reverse the rising incidence. The media have been helpful in raising the public's level of awareness.

DEPRESSION

All individuals have occasional moods of despondency and pessimism about the future. Dysphoric mood can also be secondary to physiologic changes such as menstruation, pregnancy, and medications. In pathological cases, extreme unresponsiveness to stimuli, self-deprecation, feelings of inadequacy, and hopelessness exist.

Depression is a symptom that can occur by itself (endogenous), or it can be secondary to a stressful event (exogenous).

DSM (Diagnostic and Statistical Manual of Mental Disorders) Criteria for Major Depression are:

- sad or bored mood
- diminished interest in most activities
- significant weight loss or gain
- sleep disturbance (insomnia or hypersomnia)

- motor agitation or retardation
- daily fatigue
- feelings of worthlessness or guilt
- diminished concentration
- recurrent thoughts of death or suicide

Although the same symptom criteria can be used to diagnose children and adolescents as in adults, there may be associated features that are specific for different ages (example: separation anxiety). In adolescents, irritability may mask a dysphoric mood and is considered an equivalent symptom. Medications can also cause dysphoric mood. In adolescent females, the most common pharmacologic cause of depression is birth control pills. It is frequently easier to elicit "boredom" from teens, rather than anhedonia (loss of interest in formerly pleasurable activities).

Case Study

In the early days of my career, I misdiagnosed a depression in a 15-year-old female as hypothyroidism because of my inexperience with mental health conditions. When thyroid function studies came back normal, a colleague suggested the diagnosis of depression, which was confirmed by a psychiatrist. Fortunately, the proper diagnosis was not long delayed and treatment was effective. The ending might not have been a happy one had the patient's depression and suicidal thoughts been allowed to progress unchecked.

What careful listeners we health professionals must be!

Associated Features

Major depression is equally common among prepubertal males and females, but more common in adolescent females (males tend to underreport their symptoms). The student may exhibit declining school performance (many adolescents become more symptomatic with the opening of school), may reject friends, and develop psychosomatic complaints. Morbid thoughts are common and concentration can be so impaired that depressed teens look confused. Premenstrual syndrome may worsen the picture in females.

Studies in twins give strong support to a genetic predisposition for depression (76% concordance in identical twins).

The most potent environmental factors are death of a loved one and family divorce. Certain chronic physical illnesses predispose teens to major depressive disorder: epilepsy, chronic inflammatory bowel disease, and juvenile diabetes mellitus). Anxiety disorders, conduct disorder, and attention deficit disorder sometimes co-exist.

Mania is sometimes seen between depressive episodes and is characterized by an elevated, irritable, or expansive mood manifested by restlessness, talkativeness, and grandiosity. When mania is present, a diagnosis of bipolar disorder (formerly called manic-depressive disorder) is warranted.

Two useful self-administered screening instruments (checklists) are the Beck Depression Inventory and the Weinberg Screening Affective Scale. The latter is shown in Figure 4-1, at the end of the chapter.

Treatment

Those depressive episodes whose manifestations are primarily psychological can be successfully treated with psychotherapy. When troublesome physical symptoms are present, they should be treated simultaneously. Antidepressant medication may not be necessary unless there is a recurrence or failure of psychotherapy alone.

Two commonly used antidepressants are

- imipramine (Tofranil)
- amitriptyline (Elavil)

Medication should be continued for six months and administration at school is not usually necessary. These antidepressants have a small margin of safety, and therefore should be under the control of a parent to prevent their use for suicide. If psychotherapy and an antidepressant are not effective, lithium may be added. All these treatment modalities have been shown to be superior to no treatment.

Explanation of the manifestations of depression to family, friends, and school officials puts the student's behavior in context and facilitates acceptance and minimizes possible stigma.

SUICIDE

Adolescents who attempt suicide have a greater number of negative life events and fewer personal resources and social supports than those who do not. Other factors that have a significant correlation with suicide are teen pregnancy, child abuse, and family disorganization and violence.

Adolescent suicide attempters have rates of current illness 30% to 40% greater than controls. Affective disorders (mood disorders), conduct disorders (delinquent behavior), and substance abuse are the most common psychiatric disorders associated with suicidal behavior in the young. Substance abuse has been found (either alone or with affective disorder) in more than one-third of young suicides.

Only half of completed suicides have had previous contact with a mental health professional.

Contagion Effects

Clusters of suicide in teenagers and young adults in recent years point to the role of imitation and contagion as risk factors for suicidal behavior. Contagion pathways can occur through direct or indirect knowledge of the index (primary) suicide: directly through a friend or personal acquaintance or indirectly through the media. Either way, identification of susceptible individuals with the index case is thought to underlie contagion.

The CDC (1988) has issued recommendations for community plans for the prevention and containment of suicide clusters.

Availability of Firearms

A substantial rise in firearm suicide rates has occurred since 1970 among males ages 15–24. This corresponds to large increases in the manufacture of firearms in the United States. Death by firearms is a common method of suicide, especially when the victim is intoxicated. Thus, the increasing availability of firearms and the use of alcohol among youth (the number one drug of abuse) have contributed to the increases in suicide rates. The same inference can be drawn for homicide rates.

Other Considerations

Suicidal behavior is multidetermined. Biological and cultural factors appear to play secondary roles to social factors in influencing its expression.

Figure 4-2 illustrates an adapted version of Blumenthal's model (1988) for understanding suicidal behavior.

The greatest barrier health professionals must overcome is fear of asking young people about suicidal thoughts. Talking about suicide does *not* increase suicidal acts. On the contrary, it effects two positive elements: (1) it serves as a safety valve by allowing the teen to talk about emotions (rather than internalize them), and (2) it lets the teen know that someone cares enough to ask (support system).

Unfortunately there are no satisfactory treatments for personality disorders, or disorders of impulse control, but depression can be treated successfully. Crisis hot lines and suicide prevention hot lines can be effective ways to route troubled youth into the mental health system.

Suicide is a relatively infrequent event, therefore difficult to study and predict. We are learning more about assigning weight to various risk factors, but suicidal risk assessment remains clinical for any given individual. Allowing adequate interview time for the youngster to talk (employing open-ended questions and interviewing parents and others) should enable you and the psychologist to decide who is at risk and how urgent the situation is. Maintain a high index of suspicion for suicide (especially with males) and a willingness to over-refer. Even if they are not suicidal, most troubled students can be helped by a mental health referral.

ANTISOCIAL BEHAVIOR AND VIOLENCE

What is this thing called resilience, which allows some children to resist stress and escape damage despite psychosocial adversity?

The severely physically abused child is somewhat analogous to the "barn-yard dog" who is kicked and beaten daily. A point is reached where all behaviors are pathological, maladaptive, and irreversible (sociopathic). Many of these unfortunate individuals find themselves on the streets or in jail as teens. Courts and social agencies often do not act until a law is broken or a life-threatening event has occurred. Many abused children become abusing parents, completing the cycle of violence.

Antisocial behavior and violence would all but disappear if each child had a nurturing home environment. Since society cannot provide this (primary prevention), we are left with trying to minimize exposure to and effects from abuse and neglect (secondary prevention). Strategies in this latter category include

- earlier reporting of abuse (by family members, neighbors, and others)
- a social service system staffed well enough to investigate *all* reports
- judges who are quicker to remove children from abusing, dysfunctional parents
- more alternative placements (foster homes, etc.) for children who are removed from their primary home

More generous funding of agencies is the logical starting point for more effective intervention. We have the know-how, but not the wherewithal.

Society's Influence on Child Development

Individuals depend on their culture for a coherent approach to life. Culture is the integrated pattern of human knowledge, belief, and behavior that depends on a capacity for learning and transmitting knowledge to succeeding generations. Cultures can be geographic (regional) or ethnic.

A culture provides people with a number of ready-made answers for crucial life problems. It dictates the routine relationships and social arrangements for survival needs and the protection and raising of children. In other words, it gives an entire group of people a means of coping with the world. Through communication, individuals acquire a sense of common meaning and purpose that contributes strongly to a particular way of life. This social reality is passed along through the family and educational system. It influences an individual's way of thinking and acting and can limit or enhance the type of life a person leads.

Culture is more than the external forms of clothing, food, and music. To truly understand a person's behavior, you need an awareness of the values and attitudes that have become a part of his or her mentality.

Conformity: Compliance vs. Acceptance

The psychological force that causes a person to act in accordance with the expectations of others is called *conformity*. We refer to this as social pressure or peer pressure. Although this force continues in varying degrees throughout adulthood, it is strongest in upper elementary and junior high school students (ages 10–15). A positive peer group experience for this age group is essential for healthy development. Groups and clubs that engage in risk-taking or illegal behaviors produce individuals that are ripe for gang membership. Most gangs in turn engage in antisocial and often violent behaviors. Many young people join gangs to "parent" each other when adequate parenting is absent in the home. Male gang members of 15 to 18 years of age are trying to show each other how to be "men." Macho posturing is part and parcel of gang membership, with each member trying to top the others. Drive-by shootings are often related to "initiation rites" for gang membership. Combating this disturbing mentality is an awesome undertaking.

Coping Skills

Violence (or sometimes complete withdrawal—most often in females) results from external stressors with which the individual cannot cope. Some students carry weapons to school for self-defense—not to perpetrate violence. Much violence emanates from drug trafficking controlled by adults who use juvenile "runners" because prosecution is light and the adults often cannot be linked to the juveniles. When law enforcement makes this link, the young person may be threatened, maimed, or even killed.

Teaching decision making, coping skills, and conflict resolution to young people is a long and continuous process, but the only hope of breaking the cycle of violence. Parents and schools must begin early to model conflict resolution—to demonstrate that there are ways superior to physical violence for resolving differences. The key to success is to teach students that they are in charge of their lives and can control much of their environment. Most of what happens for them depends on how they behave and react. Methods of de-escalating conflict can be practiced through role playing. The reduced stress that comes from avoiding or reducing conflict is reinforcing and contagious. It allows students to get on with more important aspects of their lives.

School nurses, because of their scientific background, can usually be more objective than other school officials in discussing the causes and effects of student behavior. You can help sort out the mildly troubled child from the truly dysfunctional one and help the latter receive proper mental health care.

While overpopulation and poverty have been blamed for the violence of inner cities, there is no absolute cause-and-effect relationship. Good parents and good schools can go a long way toward interrupting the cycle of violence.

DRUG ABUSE

Most drug abuse results from a combination of experimentation, peer pressure, and external and internal stressors. If a young person's environment causes anxiety and an illicit drug eases the pain, the gateway for abuse has been opened. These circumstances, coupled with the young person's feeling of invincibility and ignorance of addictions, has her or him well on the way to chronic abuse.

Alcohol is still the number one drug of abuse among young people. Driving while intoxicated results in the largest number of deaths in the adolescent age group.

Identifying Drug Abuse

It is axiomatic that to diagnose a problem you must suspect it. Keep a high index of suspicion for drug use. The first signs are often physical. Figure 4-3 illustrates an assessment form useful in recording the objective signs of drug use. For example, dilated pupils, rapid pulse, and talkativeness are the manifestations of stimulants such as amphetamines (speed); drowsiness, and slurred speech in the absence of an alcohol odor may mean a depressant or sedative drug is being used. Sending these recorded findings along with a referral will narrow the drug testing performed on blood, urine, or breath.

Once the drug of abuse is identified, a treatment plan can be developed. Polydrug use (alcohol plus marijuana, etc.) is hardest to treat. Any delay in referral for treatment diminishes the likelihood of a good outcome. Remember that while it may take years for an adult "social drinker" to become alcoholic, the teen can become dependent quite rapidly.

Promoting Treatment

Schools can promote the treatment of drug abusing adolescents by facilitating referrals to specialized centers and by not invoking punitive measures in first offenders who agree to treatment. It is advisable to make site visits to drug treatment centers to become familiar with their programs, especially plans for reintegrating students into the school setting.

Hopeful Trend

There has been a decrease in illegal drug use over the past decade—from 24 million users in 1979 to 11.4 million in 1992 (Kleber, 1994). Schools, particularly health educators and school nurses, play an important role in seeing that the downward trend continues. Each year a new group of at-risk youngsters enters school. Our vigorous drug abuse education efforts must not let up. Experimenting with drugs is *not* a normal part of growing up, and we must continue to send this message loudly and clearly. The drug problem will ultimately be solved at the local level, not by a federal program.

PSYCHOTHERAPY

The adolescent and his or her parents must be prepared mentally to see a psychiatrist or other mental health professional. The first step is debunking common myths (Backman 1994).

Myth 1: Talking with someone about my problems will only make them worse. (Reframed: If I get things off my chest, I'll feel better.)

Myth 2: Going to a therapist means you are crazy. (Reframed: Going to a therapist means I'm trying to help myself.)

Myth 3: No one can help me. (Reframed: I'm going to take control and find someone who can help me.)

Myth 4: I'll find out something about myself I'd rather not know. (Reframed: It doesn't mean I'm a bad person just because there are things about me that I don't like.)

Dr. Backman's excellent book, *Choosing a Therapist,* (see references at the end of this chapter) is written for secondary students and very helpful to troubled youth who are resistant to seeking mental health evaluation and treatment.

Counseling vs. Psychotherapy

Counseling is designed to provide advice and guidance for acute problems—problems such as breaking up with a boyfriend or girlfriend or having a fight with a parent.

Psychotherapy is geared to getting at the root of long-standing problems such as chronic sadness, drinking too much, or having irrational fears. The person in psychotherapy is not going just for advice or answers, but for understanding. This process takes longer than counseling. Psychotherapy can be provided by psychiatrists, psychologists, and certain types of social workers and master's level counselors with mental health training.

Types of Psychotherapy

Formally defined, psychotherapy is the application of specialized techniques to the treatment of mental disorders or to the problems of everyday adjustment. Examples of the techniques used are psychodrama, psychoanalysis, directive and nondirective counseling, in-depth interview, suggestion, conditioning, and interpretation. All involve close communication between therapist and client, in which the client discusses his or her most intimate experiences without fear of moral judgment. The goal of all psychotherapy is to encourage understanding of a problem.

Types of psychotherapy include

- *Psychoanlaysis*—Adults, rather than teens, usually go into psychoanalysis, since the main focus is on helping one understand the past and how basic character has been formed. With young people, this technique may be used when their development has been slowed or arrested in some way. The basic method of psychoanalysis is "free association," in which the patient is encouraged to discuss everything that comes into his or her mind. Usually, two or more years are required for adequate psychoanalysis.
- *Psychodynamic psychotherapy*—This is the most common form of psychotherapy. Psychodynamic therapy focuses on conflicts in one's personal life. Although it draws on the past, that is not the main focus. It is geared to help individuals deal with a current situation by focusing on interpersonal relationships and how they influence behavior positively and negatively.
- *Behavioral therapy*—Here the focus is to change unwanted behaviors, such as phobias, anxiety, and tobacco addiction. Specific techniques used include relaxation exercises, desensitization, behavior modification, and hypnosis.
- *Cognitive therapy*—Emotional problems are thought to come from distorted and self-defeating ways of thinking. The goal of cognitive therapy is to help one see the role that thoughts play in behavior and feelings. Through therapy, the person learns to identify negative thoughts and replace them with more realistic ones. The theory is that changing thought patterns will change feelings and behavior.

SCHOOL NURSE ROLE

You can go a long way toward helping the adolescent solve his or her problems by being a nonjudgmental listener, and when appropriate, referring to specialized mental health professionals. Figures 4-4 and 4-5 are forms that can be used to obtain parent permission and request psychiatric consultation.

As a "sounding board," you provide a reality check for the student and help separate major from minor problems, and symptoms from their underlying cause. Problems that seem overwhelming to the isolated teen will often shrink into perspective in the presence of a sympathetic ear.

Keep your antennae up!

SUMMARY

Human behavior is the complex result of a number of forces acting on the individual. Without getting bogged down in the nature vs. nurture conundrum, it is clear that adolescents, much more than adults, are subject to environmental influences. Understanding the teenage student means understanding his or her environment and sorting out the positive and negative influences.

Sometimes a solution lies in removing the young person from the negative influence (avoidance of a drug-using peer group). At other times a solution to a problem is found by teaching the adolescent useful coping skills (conflict resolution; stress reduction). Always, it means building on the strengths and aspirations of the individual and maximizing the support of important peers and adults. The greatest challenge comes when these support systems are weak or absent.

REFERENCES

1. Atkins, D. "Clinical Spectrum of Anorexia Nervosa in Children." *Developmental and Behavioral Pediatrics* 14(4):211–216, 1993.

2. Backman, M. *Choosing a Therapist: A Young Person's Guide to Counselling and Psychotherapy.* New York: Rosen Publishing Group, 1994.

3. Cohall. A. "Teen Violence: The Search for Solutions." *Contemporary Pediatrics* (November), 1991.

4. De Maso, D. "Depressive Disorders and Suicidal Intent in Adolescent Suicide Attempters." *Developmental and Behavioral Pediatrics* 15(2):74–77, 1994.

   — Programs for the Prevention of Suicide Among Adolescents & Young Adults, *Morbidity & Mortality Weekly Report* (Centers for Disease Control, Atlanta), 43 (RR-6): 3–17, 1994.

   — CDC Recommendations for a Community Plan for the Prevention & Containment of Suicide Clusters. *Morbidity and Mortality Weekly Report* 37 (5–8):1–8, 1988.

5. — *DSM-IV Draft Criteria.* Washington, DC: American Psychiatric Association, 1993.

6. Emslie, G. "Depressive Symptoms by Self-Report in Adolescence." *Journal of Child Neurology* 5:114–121, 1990.

7. Goldenring, J. "Getting into Adolescent Heads." *Contemporary Pediatrics* (July 1988): 75–90.

8. Good, W. *Psychiatry Made Ridiculously Simple.* Miami, Fla: MedMaster, Inc., 1992.

9. Kemph, J. "Treatment of Aggressive Children with Clonidine." *Journal of the American Academy of Child and Adolescent Psychiatry* 32(3):577–581, 1993.

10. Kleber, H. "Our Current Approach to Drug Abuse." *New England Journal of Medicine* 330(5):361–365, 1994.

11. Kramer, P. *Listening to Prozac.* New York: Viking, 1993.

12. Matier, K. "Methylphenidate Response in Aggressive and Nonaggressive Children." *J. Am. Acad. Child Asolesc. Psychiatry* 31(2):219–225, 1992.

13. Millon, T. (ed.). *Contemporary Directions in Psychopathology.* New York: Guilford Press, 1986.

14. Puskar, Kathryn. "Adolescent Mental Health: Collaboration Among Psychiatric Mental Health Nurses and School Nurses." *Journal of School Health* 60(2):69–71, 1990.

15. Rutter, M. "Resilience: Some Conceptual Considerations." *Contemporary Pediatrics* 11:36–48, 1994.

16. Shorter, E. *From the Mind into the Body.* New York: Free Press (Macmillan), 1994.

17. Singer. M. *Handbook for Screening Adolescents at Psychological Risk.* New York: Lexington Books (Macmillan), 1993.

18. Swanson, N. "Identifying Potential Dropouts. *Journal of School Nursing* 10(2):22–27, 1994.

19. — "Violence-Related Attitudes and Behaviors of High School Students." *Morbidity & Mortality Weekly Report* (Centers for Disease Control, Atlanta). 42(40):773–777, 1993.

20. Weinberg, W. "Weinberg Screening Affective Scale." *Journal of Child Neurology* 3:294–296, 1988.

Figure 4-1

WEINBERG SCREENING AFFECTIVE SCALE
(SHORT FORM)

Instructions: We would like to ask you some serious questions. We want to know how you feel about yourself. If you agree with the statement, circle yes. If you do not agree with the statement, circle no. We consider your answers very important.

1. I will try to give my honest feelings on these questions.	Yes	No
2. I can't concentrate on my work.	Yes	No
3. I feel lonely too much of the time.	Yes	No
4. I don't want to go to school anymore.	Yes	No
5. It seems like some part of my body always hurts me.	Yes	No
6. People are always talking about me when I'm not there.	Yes	No
7. I have too many bad moods.	Yes	No
8. I don't have fun playing with my friends anymore.	Yes	No
9. It's hard to fall asleep and that bothers me.	Yes	No
10. I can't do anything right.	Yes	No
11. I feel too tired to play.	Yes	No
12. I daydream too much in school.	Yes	No
13. I wish I were dead.	Yes	No
14. My answers are how I have been feeling most of the time.	Yes	No
15. These answers represent my honest feelings.	Yes	No

0-3 Probably no further assessment necessary
4-6 Evaluation by school psychologist
7+ (or yes on #13) Immediate referral

Figure 4-2

THRESHOLD MODEL FOR SUICIDAL BEHAVIOR*

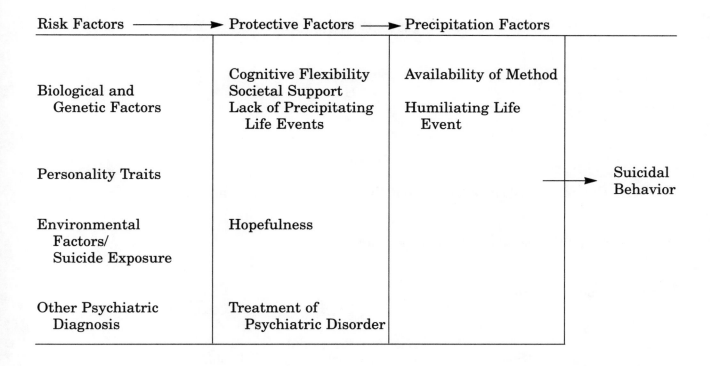

*(Adapted from Blumenthal, *Journal of Adolescent Psychiatry 27*: 313–322, 1988)

Figure 4-3

ASSESSMENT FORM FOR SUSPECTED CHEMICAL USE
(Confidential Information - For Medical Personnel Only)

Demographic Data

Date:
Time:

Name: DOB:
Address: School ID#:
Parents: Home Phone #:
School: Work Phone #:
Grade:

History

Student's Comments: (Write exactly what the student says in regard to this situation)

Administrator's Comments: (Attendance, grades, behavior)

Other Significant History:

Physical Assessment
(See Drug and Alcohol Abuse: Everyone's Problem)

Vital Signs: B/P _____ Pulse _____ Resp. _____ Temp. _____ Wt. _____
General Appearance: (Describe)
Visual Acuity: (At time of assessment)   O.D. _____   O.S. _____
Pupil Size: (In mm)

| 1 | 2 | 3 | 4 | 5 | 6 | 7 | 8 |

Circle the appropriate description and comment if abnormal.

	Right	Left
Pupil Reaction: (Comments)	Normal Sluggish Fixed	Normal Sluggish Fixed
Nose: (Comments)	Normal Rhinorrhea Residue	Mucosal Color Septal Perforation
Mouth: (Comments)	Normal Odor Buccal Mucosa	Lips Raw Dry Cracked

Figure 4-3 (Continued)

	Right	Left
Arm Strength: (Comments)	Normal Increased Decreased	Normal Increased Decreased

	Right	Left
Leg Strength: (Comments)	Normal Increased Decreased	Normal Increased Decreased

Skin: (Comments)	Normal
	Puncture
	   Wounds
	Scars
		Lacerations
		Bruises
		Color
		   Pale
		   Flushed

Lungs/Chest: (Describe breath sounds, i.e., rales, rhonchi, wheezes)
(Comments)

Mental Status: (Comments)

Cognitive: (Affect, Hallucinations, Illusions, Orientation, Somnolent, Confused, Incomplete Sentences, Inappropriate Words, Lethargy, Poor Perception of Time and Distance, Increase in Alertness, Decrease in Alertness)

Behavior: (Paranoia, Anxiety, Depression, Hyperactive, Euphoric, Breakdown of Inhibitions, Increase in Appetite, Excitation, Decrease in Appetite, Drowsiness, Relaxation)

Coordination: (Test Romberg, Finger-Nose, Finger-Finger, One Foot Stand)

Other Significant Factors:

Assessment Statement: (State your assessment of the student's status and recommendation for follow-up.)

Outcome: (Follow-up)
Medical: (Was student referred? Was referral completed?)

Other: (Administrative, Parental)

(Attach this form to Medical Referral/Follow-up Form (H16) if medical referral is made.)

Figure 4-4

PARENT PERMISSION FORM FOR PSYCHIATRIC CONSULTATION

Name_____ Birthdate _____ School _____

Is your child under the care of a doctor? _____ Yes _____No

If yes, may we contact the doctor about your child? _____Yes _____No

Name and agency or address of doctor_____

Name *Agency or address*

List all prescription medications that your child is taking:

Medicine	Dose	Time of day taken	Given at home or school?	For what problem?
_____	_____	_____	_____	_____
_____	_____	_____	_____	_____
_____	_____	_____	_____	_____
_____	_____	_____	_____	_____
_____	_____	_____	_____	_____

Other comments:

I give permission for my child to be interviewed at school by school district physicians or consultants. If medicine is needed to help my child to learn at school, I give permission for the medicine to be prescribed, and I will help to see that it is given. I understand that there will be no charge for the psychiatric consultation, but I will be expected to purchase any necessary medication. I understand that I will be contacted by the physician or nurse practitioner before the medicine is prescribed or changed. I understand that I will be notified of my child's appointment with the doctor, and I will attempt to be present at the school for that appointment.

_____   _____
Date   *Parent's signature*

AUTORIZACION DEL PADRE PARA UNA CONSULTA PSIQUIATRICA

Nombre _____ Fecha de Nacimiento _____ Escuela _____

¿Está su hijo/a bajo los cuidados de un doctor? _____ Sí _____ No

Si es Sí, ¿podemos ponernos en contacto con el doctor de su hijo? _____ Sí _____ No

Nombre de la agencia o dirección del doctor_____

                                                Nombre   *Agencia o dirección*

Mencione todos los medicamentos que se le han recetado a su hijo/a:

Medicina	Dosis	Hora en que debe tomarse	¿En la casa o en la escuela?	¿Para qué tipo de problema?

Otros comentarios:

Doy mi consentimiento para que mi hijo sea entrevistado en la escuela por doctores o especialistas del Distrito Escolar. Si se necesita algún tipo de medicina que pueda ser beneficiosa para mi hijo en su aprendizaje en la escuela, doy mi consentimiento para que se recete dicha medicina y cooperaré asegurándome de que lo tome. Entiendo que no pagaré por la consulta médica pero es mi responsabilidad comprar cualquier medicina que sea necesaria. También entiendo que un doctor o enfermera se pondrá en contacto conmigo antes que se decida recetar o cambiar la medicina a mi hijo/a. Entiendo que se me comunicará acerca de las citas de mi hijo/a con el doctor y haré todo lo posible por estar presente en la escuela para dicha cita.

_____   _____
Fecha   *Firma del Padre / Tutor*

Figure 4-5

REQUEST FOR PSYCHIATRIC CONSULTATION

Student's Name _____ D.O.B _____

Date _____ School _____ Requested by _____

Suspected Med/psychiatric diagnosis _____

Parent's name _____ Date of permission _____

Medical

Summary and current status of pertinent medical findings, tests, reports, prenatal and developmental history, current and past medications (dosage, who prescribed, date), results of prior consultations, and medical care including names of doctors and agencies.

Family Data

Family composition, any recent significant events, family history of mental or emotional disorder.

School

Specific concerns regarding behavior, academic level, instructional arrangement; describe time of day and context when behavior problem occurs; describe any time periods during the day when student is unsupervised.

Summary of Test Data

Include any significant findings from academic and/or psychological assessment reports.

PSYCHIATRIST'S SUMMARY OF FINDINGS / DIAGNOSES

PSYCHIATRIST'S RECOMMENDATIONS

To school:

To parents:

_____   _____
Signature   Date

CHAPTER 5

GAY AND LESBIAN YOUTH

Chapter 5

GAY AND LESBIAN YOUTH

Nature never rhymes her children, nor makes two
men alike.

Ralph Waldo Emerson, 1844

REAL STORIES

I knew I was different from the 7th grade. My classmates had gone girl crazy
and I could care less. Wasn't there anyone else like me? I kept my secret and
played the game, but I felt dishonest and alone.

Jeff, age 16

Telling my parents was a traumatic experience. My father exploded; my
mother cried. They felt angry and guilty. I felt hurt. It was a bad, bad scene.
Eventually things smoothed out some, but our relationship was never the same.
It was different with my sister—she accepted my gayness right away.

Rosa, age 17

When heterosexuals are asked, "When did you decide to be straight?" they
respond: "I didn't have to. I always was." Gays "always were," too, but they have
to think about it a little more because of society's negative messages. Few visi-
ble role models exist to say "you're okay, too," so it takes gays longer to understand their sexual orientation.

FROM KINSEY TO THE PRESENT

The Kinsey Report of 1953 found that few people were exclusively heterosexual
or homosexual. Dr. Kinsey created a seven-point scale to depict sexual orientation as a continuum (the two extremes, 0 and 6, being exclusively heterosexual

or homosexual). Those persons with equally balanced feelings or experiences fall in the middle and are termed bisexual. Kinsey's figures for homosexuality were: female 5%, male 10%.

More recently, Storms (1980) stated that sexual orientation should be thought of two-dimensionally, that is individuals should be rated separately on heterosexual and homosexual attraction. Thus, a person could be high on both, low on both, or high on one scale and low on the other. *This approach eliminates the concept that bisexuality is a weak mixture of the two extremes—that one form of sexual expression "crowds out" another.* See the end of the chapter for "Two-dimensional scale of sexual orientation," Figure 5-1, which illustrates this.

WHAT CAUSED HIM TO BE GAY OR HER TO BE LESBIAN?

Parents always ask this question. Young people want to know, too. There are a number of theories, but no one really knows. The bulk of evidence strongly suggests that a person is born that way. A choice is not made. Parents sometimes worry that they caused it. Some church officials say it's the devil or personal choice. The scientific community subscribes to neither of these concepts. Homosexuality just is.

Psychiatrists have concluded that homosexuality is not a disease to be cured. The term was removed from the *Third Edition of the Diagnostic and Statistical Manual* (American Psychiatric Association) in 1974 (except for its ego-dystonic form). In the Fourth Edition (1994), the term homosexuality does not even appear in the index.

Current research is exploring brain anatomy and endocrine metabolism for differences between heterosexual and homosexual individuals.

HOW MANY ARE THERE?

Estimates of the number of gays range from 1% to 10%. In the United States there are 249 million people (1990 census), which means between 2.5 and 25 million people are gay. It's certainly not rare. Nearly 26% of Americans are under 18 years of age (64 million). A conservative estimate of 5% gay or lesbian means at least 3.2 million teens belong to this group.

DEVIANT SEXUAL BEHAVIOR

Some homosexual youth are not troubled by their sexual orientation; they are comfortable with their assigned gender (what's on their birth certificate) and their same-sex attraction. Many, however, have difficulty dealing with society's non-acceptance. As previously stated, homosexuality does not appear in the *DSM*, except in its ego-dystonic form. There are, however, a group of sexual deviations that do appear in the *DSM* and thus represent pathologies warranting mental health diagnoses. For adolescents, the major one is *gender identity disorder* (GID).

Gender Identity Disorder

The criteria for diagnosis of GID are:
For females:

A. Intense distress about being a girl, a stated desire to be a boy, and

B. Either 1 or 2
    1. Aversion to feminine clothing
    2. Repudiation of female anatomic structures

For males:

A. Intense distress about being a boy, a desire to be a girl, and

B. Either 1 or 2
    1. Preoccupation with female activities and dress
    2. Repudiation of male anatomic structures

If these criteria persist for at least two years, a diagnosis of transsexualism is made. Generally there is a moderate to severe co-existing personality disturbance. Frequently the person experiences anxiety that he or she attributes to the inability to be in the role of the desired sex.

Paraphilias

The paraphilias are characterized by sexual arousal in response to objects or situations that are unusual and interfere with affectionate sexual activity. Examples include exhibitionism, fetishism (including cross-dressing fetishism), sexual masochism or sadism, voyeurism, and pedophilia. The last example involves sexual activity with a prepubescent child. This, of course, is a criminal offense and taboo in virtually all cultures in the United States. In terms of arrests, male heterosexuals are the primary perpetrators of this crime. Unfortunately, homosexuals are all perceived as pedophiles—preying on children—by society largely because the media more widely publicize homosexual pedophilia. (See the following glossary.) The most common scenario of pedophilia is the abuse of a female child by an adult male relative.

SORTING THROUGH THE TERMINOLOGY MAZE

Before proceeding it will be important to understand a few additional terms.

Bisexuality: equal, or near equal, attraction to persons of the same and opposite sex.

Coming out: discovering one's homosexual orientation and disclosing it to others.

Dysfunctional family: one whose members behave in maladaptive ways that stifle healthy development of children; examples are uncontrolled rage or violence, denial of addictive behavior, inconsistent discipline, alcoholism, and/or severe physical abuse.

Ego-dystonic homosexuality: unwanted or distressing same sex attraction; may represent confusion about or failure to accept one's sexual orientation.

Ego-syntonic homosexuality: acceptance of and comfort with one's sexual orientation.

Gay: homosexual; can refer to both males and females, but increasingly used to refer to men.

Gender role: an individual's characteristics or personality traits that are culturally defined as masculine or feminine.

Heterosexual assumption: the assumption that everyone is heterosexual, as with issues of dating, marriage, and having children; also known as heterosexism.

Homophobia: dislike or fear of homosexuals as a group.

Homosexual myths: false beliefs about gay men and lesbians, such as "homosexuals hate and fear the opposite sex."

Homosexuality: erotic attraction, predisposition, or sexual behavior between individuals of the same sex, especially postpuberty.

Kinsey scale: a seven-point scale developed by Alfred Kinsey to describe a continuum of sexual orientation. The scale ranges from exclusive heterosexuality to exclusive homosexuality, with gradations between. Most people are located between the two extremes.

Lesbian: a female homosexual.

Paraphilia: sexual practices that are legally or socially prohibited. Examples include pedophilia, sexual masochism, voyeurism, and transvestic fetishism. (The presence of these behaviors is pathological and warrants a mental health diagnosis.)

Pedophilia: sexual activity of an adult with a prepubertal child; the adult is at least 16 years of age and at least five years older than the child.

Sex: biological status as a female or male; same as gender.

Sexual identity: an individual's sense of self as male or female.

Sexual orientation: the attraction of an individual to persons of the same, or opposite sex, or both, that is homosexual, heterosexual, or bisexual. Same as sexual preference.

Transsexual: a person whose sexual identity (male or female) is different from his or her biological gender. Example: A man who describes himself as a woman trapped in a man's body; transsexuals may desire sex-change operations.

Transvestite: cross-dresser; a person who wears clothing of the opposite biological gender—most often a man who dresses in women's clothing. (There are also heterosexual cross-dressers.)

THE COMING-OUT PROCESS

Gay males begin to suspect that they might be homosexual at an average age of 17; lesbians at an average age of 18. Many young people suspect this difference at a much younger age—some claim 13 or even younger. At whatever age that earliest suspicion of difference occurs, the homosexual identity evolves over an extended period of time, against a backdrop of stigma. Four stages of homosexual realization are as follows:

Stage I—*Sensitization.* Before puberty one may come to understand the meaning of the term *homosexual,* but it is not generally seen as personally relevant, although there may be vague feelings of "being different."

Stage II—*Identity Confusion.* Gay males and lesbians begin to personalize homosexuality during adolescence as they relate their feelings to their understanding of the definition of homosexuality. Initially this is not in concert with previously held self-images.

Stage III—*Identity Assumption.* In late adolescence (or even later) the individual accepts himself or herself as a homosexual. They usually associate with other gays and experiment sexually as well as explore the homosexual subculture. Males achieve this stage, on the average, between 19 and 21 years. Lesbians reach homosexual self-definitions between 21 and 23 years (Schafer, 1976).

Stage IV—*Commitment.* In this final stage, individuals adopt homosexuality as a way of life and disclose themselves to others. Entering a same-sex love relationship marks the onset of commitment. This stage may range from the late 20s to 30s for both females and males.

True bisexuals may take the longest to complete Stage II because they assume that sexual orientation is an "either-or" proposition.

COUNSELING GAY AND LESBIAN YOUTH

Sexual Reorientation Therapy

Some parents, church counselors, and other professionals will suggest that a young person can be reprogrammed to be heterosexual. However, most authorities believe that attempts at reorientation therapy are unsuccessful and should not be undertaken. Even Freud understood homosexuality to be compatible not only with normal psychological function but also with superior mental and moral qualities.

Helping Teens to Know Themselves

"Am I gay?" Most young people who ask this question are. A few are not.

The first step toward getting on with life is for each individual to answer the question honestly—without qualification or rationalization. When a student has expressed concern about sexual orientation, the self-administered questionnaire illustrated in Figure 5-2 can be a starting point for dialogue. In some communities school nurses will want to obtain parental permission before obtaining the information in this questionnaire.

Finding Someone to Trust

It is virtually impossible for an isolated individual to grow up well adjusted and happy; keeping homosexuality to oneself for too long is unhealthy. It's hard to concentrate on school or work. One philosopher said, "Hiding your essential being is one of life's greatest tortures." Eventually someone must know, and the student may come to you for guidance.

Specific Strategies

When a young person has come to grips with the probability that he or she is homosexual (this *is* self-determined—never "diagnosed" externally), the strategies that follow can be used to determine a course of action. Suggest that the young person

1. Reflect on the answers to the check-list in Figure 5-2. If the answers strongly indicate that the student is homosexual, he or she can be helped in taking steps toward self-acceptance.
2. Seek out a confidant. He or she can set a goal of one or two months to find someone to talk to. Many lesbians and gay males find it easier to talk to a female friend—someone who already values them as individuals.
3. Be prepared for rejection, but keep searching for a sympathetic ear.
4. Share his or her concerns and feelings with the confidant. Using the person as a sounding board will help the young person to check her or his self-perceptions.

Advise young people to move slowly in acting on their homosexuality—not to hide it, but to choose carefully the person to whom they "come out." Confiding in the wrong individual can lead to gossip at school and it can be a terrible thing to experience. "Fag" and "dyke" jokes hurt. Prudence is the best approach for gay youth.

As stated in strategy 2, advise a teen to select a good friend of either sex and test the waters. Is she or he intelligent and compassionate? Does that friend respect the person? Have confidences been kept in the past? If the answers to these questions are yes, it is usually safe. It should be presented as a matter-of-fact part of the young person's whole being without apology or dramatization.

If the news has been received in a positive or neutral fashion, the student should probably let it rest for a while—allow the friend to digest and think about what has been said. If the news has been received very negatively—or with disgust—tell the young person to write that individual off her or his friendship list. This aversion is probably too deep-seated to overcome. If the friend is only mildly shocked, have your student pursue these feelings. Say, "Chances are, if he or she knows you well and respects you, you'll be able to bring your friend around."

Once a young person has established the acceptance and trust of a friend, the friend can help decide how to break the news to parents and siblings.

TELLING PARENTS AND OTHERS

Somehow mothers have a way of knowing. It is best to start with Mother. She can, given time, become an ally in breaking the news to Dad.

Fathers seem more inclined to deny the facts. If feelings have been shared with siblings, they may help when parents are told; their acceptance will be an eye-opener. Here again, however, the student should be cautioned that acceptance is not guaranteed.

Sharing with other adults, relatives, and classmates need not be done right away—or ever. But if asked, they should remember that honesty is best unless there is an overriding reason not to be truthful.

WHEN THINGS AREN'T GOING WELL

When the teen has come out to a few people and it is not being well received, stop and ask why. Often it has to do with certain myths about homosexuals. Dr. Margaret Schneider (*Often Invisible*, 1988) has catalogued the myths that mark homophobia.

Myth 1: Homosexuals are fundamentally different from heterosexuals.

Myth 2: Homosexuals hate and fear the opposite sex.

Myth 3: Homosexuals act like the opposite sex and want to be the opposite sex.

Myth 4: Homosexuals are excessively sexual.

Myth 5: Homosexuals are threats to others. They prey on heterosexual adults and children for sexual gratification and for recruiting.

Myth 6: Homosexuals are failures. They turn to the same sex because they cannot find or maintain relationships with the opposite sex.

Myth 7: Homosexuals and their relationships are neurotic and unstable.

Myth 8: Homosexuality is chosen.

Even in the absence of homophobia, the "heterosexual assumption" causes problems for high school students.

To be prepared for the worst that may happen, have students complete the chart in Figure 5-3, "Positive Responses to Rejection."

If the telling of friends, siblings, and parents has gone poorly, the gay student may not feel equipped to deal with it alone. Often an objective professional—one with no preinvested emotions—can smooth the path through homophobic reactions. The choice of a professional will depend on the school and community. It will cost nothing, financially or emotionally, to talk to a school psychologist, counselor, or nurse. Most will not judge, but will help the young person consider options carefully. They may also suggest a community agency, some of which will see minors without parents' being present, at least for one or two visits. The clergy are a mixed group when it comes to gay youth. While some acknowledge and work with gays, others may have a negative view of homosexuality. It is important to know which group a member of the clergy is in before referring a young person.

SELLING SELF

As stated earlier, there is more to homosexuality than sex. Each person is much more than her or his sexual orientation. Ask these young people to identify their talents and strengths. Help them to sort through their thinking by completing the lists in Figure 5-4. *Example:* "I admire honesty, hard work, compassion, open-mindedness, optimism, sense of humor, flexibility, good grooming, self-discipline, and friendliness. Their opposites are the traits I dislike in other people."

Now, have the students pick out their two best points and encourage them to make sure others know about them. Say: "Sell yourself!" They should avoid physical characteristics, such as "good looking"; rather, they should list intangibles that most people would admire and respect.

By demonstrating the worth of the whole person, you can help the young person see that sexuality is only a part of each person—and in everyday life, a small part, just as it is with heterosexuals. Persuade young people not to dwell exclusively on the fact that they are gay or lesbian.

WELL FAMILIES AND SICK FAMILIES

The ideal all-American family does not exist. Fortunately, families don't have to be perfect for their children to develop a healthy self-image. Reasonably normal growth and development can take place in children if a few basics are provided beyond food, clothing, and shelter. According to Isensee (1991) these are

- dependable nurturing
- unconditional love
- empathy
- acceptance and recognition

If these needs are met, children almost always develop a positive self-image—a sense that they are loved for who they are and not for what they can provide for parents. When these conditions are met, children don't have to "prove" themselves to feel worthy. They are free to explore talents and dreams. A gay boy or lesbian girl can express an emerging sexual orientation in an environment of support.

Families who fail to provide these four basic ingredients stifle the healthy growth of their children. Such families are referred to as *dysfunctional*. They may range from overly rigid to chaotic, but all have in common ignoring or discounting a child's emotions.

Isensee's characteristics of dysfunctional families are

- rigidity
- trust violating
- intrusive
- stereotypical gender roles
- inconsistent/mixed messages
- isolated/secretive
- poor communication
- suppression of feelings
- uncontrolled rage/violence
- denial of addictive behavior
- scapegoating
- children given adult responsibilities
- chaotic environment

No dysfunctional family will have all of these characteristics.

Growing up gay in a homophobic culture can be similar to growing up in a dysfunctional family, even without abusive parents. *Most families don't consider the possibility that a child might be gay.* This absence of parental understanding experienced by so many gay youths appears to those youths to resemble the emotional neglect of abusive parents.

In rare cases the young person is better off out of the home—particularly if he or she has been kicked out by a parent. Others run away to avoid physical or emotional harm.

KEEPING A JOURNAL

One of the best ways to identify challenges and their solutions is to keep a journal or diary. Writing things down separates the big issues from the minor ones; it helps clarify thinking. Journal entries don't have to be made daily; twice a week is a good frequency for a high school student. One journal keeper has said: "I never know what I really think about a subject until I write it down; I'm often surprised."

Once major challenges have been catalogued, tell students to review their talents and strengths, and decide on solutions or goals for meeting these challenges. Each month, they re-read what is written and modify goals as needed. Most are pleased with the sense of direction this gives. Say, "Don't be too hard on yourself if some of your goals aren't met quickly; most will take time. What you write in your journal will be for your eyes only, so keep it in a safe place and don't put your name on it. You may even want to use code for certain words or people."

REVIEW OF STRATEGIES

1. Begin a journal or diary.
2. Tell a close friend you are gay.
3. Tell a sibling you are gay.
4. Tell your mother you are gay.
5. Tell your father you are gay.
6. Consider telling significant others.
7. Consult a professional if things aren't going well.
8. Continue your journal for at least six months.

The order of these strategies is one that works best for most young gays and lesbians. Some situations may call for a different order. Consider what will be best for the individual.

FINAL THOUGHTS

Bisexuality

If young people think they might be bisexual, the possibilities are that

1. they are bisexual
2. they are not totally comfortable with being lesbian or gay
3. they have had an isolated homosexual experience
4. it is "in" to be bisexual

Homosexuality a Misnomer

The term *homosexuality* is an unfortunate and inaccurate term for gays and lesbians—unfortunate because it doesn't describe the whole person.

Heterosexuals understand that there is more to them than sexuality, but many won't admit it's true for gays as well. Think of all the interests and aspirations teens have. Most are interesting and well-rounded. The only way to achieve reasonable happiness is to pursue many interests—after dealing with the part that is sexual.

Surviving

Why is there so much prejudice against gays?

Humans seem to prefer sameness, and develop a dislike or mistrust of people who are different; not only gays. Many countries still treat women and minorities as second class citizens. Diversity is more interesting and productive; it is not clear why some societies take so long to discover it.

Some young people will say, "It's all so depressing," or "I'm not a courageous person." Tell them to remember the many things that have changed because of gay people—Michelangelo, Leonardo daVinci, Sappho, Oscar Wilde, James Baldwin, Gertrude Stein, Walt Whitman, Martina Navratilova, Greg Louganis & Barney Frank. Tell them we never know whose name will be added to the list next.

SUMMARY

Parents and professionals have a mission to help young people develop into well-adjusted, productive adults. Professionals need not endorse behaviors of concern demonstrated by young people; none of us would condone sexual promiscuity, drug abuse, driving while intoxicated, or any other behavior that puts a young person at risk. Nevertheless, if we are, in fact, the helping professionals we claim to be, we must put aside our personal biases and begin to assist young people where they are. If we cannot do this with a particular problem, whether it be teen pregnancy or homosexuality, then we must step aside and let someone else extend the helping hand.

You can use the strategies presented in this chapter in counseling teens with questions regarding sexual orientation. All our youth are worth an equal investment of resources and energy, and the 10% incidence figure for gay and lesbian youth holds up in most comprehensive high schools. School officials can no longer hide behind the statement, "We don't have any of those here." You can work with counselors, psychologists, and social workers; lead the way to becoming approachable. See Figure 5-5 "Homosexuality and Adolescence" (American Academy of Pediatrics, 1983).

REFERENCES

1. Alyson, Sasha (ed.). *Young, Gay & Proud!* Boston: Alyson Publications, 1991.

2. Anderson, John: School Climate for Gay and Lesbian Students and Staff Members. *Phi Delta Kappan,* October, 1994.

3. Borhek, Mary. *Coming Out to Parents.* Cleveland: Pilgrim Press, 1983.

4. Borhek, Mary. *My Son Eric.* New York: Pilgrim Press, 1979.

5. Cohen, Susan, and Daniel Cohen. *When Someone You Know Is Gay.* New York: Dell/Laurel Leaf, 1989. (Written for heterosexual teens to promote understanding of gays.)

6. Cormier, Sid. *Am I Normal?* New York: Carrol and Graf, 1993.

7. Duplecham, Larry. *Blackbird.* New York: St. Martin's Press, 1986 (Fiction).

8. Fairchild, Betty. *Now That You Know—What Every Parent Should Know About Homosexuality.* N.Y., Harcourt-Brace (Harvest), 1979. (Recommend this to parents.)

9. Finnegan, Dana, and Emily McNally. *Dual Identities.* Center City: MN: Hazelden, 1988.

10. Forward, Susan. *Toxic Parents.* New York: Bantam Books, 1990.

11. Friedman, Richard: Homosexuality. *New England Journal of Medicine,* 331(14): 923–930, 1994.

12. Harbeck, Karen. *Coming Out of the Classroom Closet.* New York: Harrington Park Press (Haworth), 1992.

13. Herdt, Gilbert (ed.). *Gay & Lesbian Youth.* New York: Harrington Park Press, 1989.

14. Herdt, Gilbert. *Children of Horizons: How Gay and Lesbian Teens Are Leading a New Way Out of the Closet.* Boston: Beacon Press, 1993.

15. Heron, Ann (ed.). *One Teenager in Ten.* Boston: Alyson Publications. 1983. (Coming out stories by gay teens.)

16. Isensee, Rik. *Growing Up Gay in a Dysfunctional Family.* New York: Prentice Hall (Parkside Recovery Book), 1991.

17. Marcus, Eric. *Is It a Choice?* San Francisco: Harper, 1993.

18. O'Neill, Craig, and Kathleen Ritter. *Coming Out Within.* San Francisco: Harper, Collins, 1992.

19. Rench, Janice. *Understanding Sexual Identity: A Book for Gay Teens and Their Friends.* Minneapolis: Learner Publications, 1990.

20. Saverman, T. H. *Read This Before Coming Out to Your Parents.* Pamphlet from Parents and Friends of Lesbians and Gays (P-FLAG), Washington, DC, 1984.

21. Schneider, Margaret. *Often Invisible.* Toronto, Canada: Central Toronto Youth Services, 1988.

22. Siegel, Stanley. *Uncharted Lives.* New York: Dutton (Penguin), 1994.

23. Singer, B. L. *Gay and Lesbian Stats.* New York: The New Press, 1994.

24. Sullivan, Harry. *The Psychiatric Interview.* New York: W. W. Norton, 1970.

25. Weinberg, George. *Society and the Healthy Homosexual.* Boston: Alyson Publications, 1991.

26. *You Are Not Alone: National Lesbian, Gay and Bisexual Youth Organization Directory.* New York: Hetrick-Martin Institute, 1993.

Figure 5-1

TWO-DIMENSIONAL SCALE OF SEXUAL ORIENTATION
(AFTER STORMS, 1980)

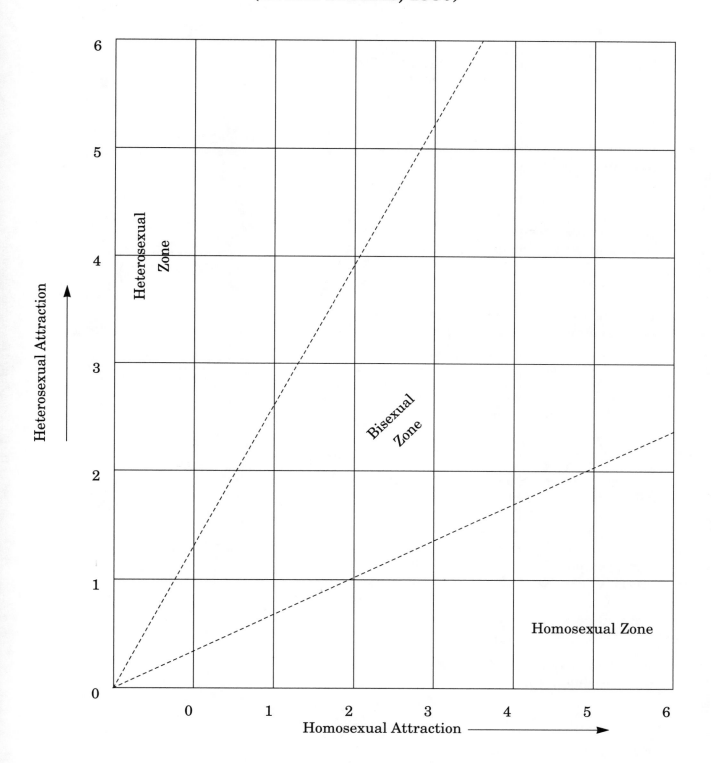

Figure 5-2

SEXUAL ORIENTATION QUESTIONNAIRE

	No	Often	Sometimes
1. Have you been criticized for not conforming to male or female role expectations?	_____	_____	_____
2. Do you have warm, physical feelings toward individuals of your own sex?	_____	_____	_____
3. Do you act on these feelings? (touching, writing notes, etc.)	_____	_____	_____
4. Have you experienced more than mutual masturbation with a same-sex friend?	_____	_____	_____
5. Do you have dreams of close physical contact with a same-sex partner?	_____	_____	_____
6. Do you have romantic fantasies about film or music stars of your gender?	_____	_____	_____
7. Have you put off having dates with the opposite sex? (Or had them but not enjoyed them?)	_____	_____	_____
8. Would you like to "live happily ever after" with a person of your own sex?	_____	_____	_____
9. For any "often" answers above, did you feel a strong need to conceal your thoughts or actions?	_____	_____	_____

If you have two or more "often" answers, consider the possibility that you are gay.

Figure 5-3

POSITIVE RESPONSES TO REJECTION

Complete the chart according to feelings, changes, and responses you might experience if these people in your life failed to accept your homosexuality.

	YOUR FEELINGS	CHANGES IN YOUR LIFE	POSITIVE RESPONSES
Friend			
Sister or Brother			
Parent			
Grandparent			

Figure 5-4

SELLING YOURSELF

Personality traits I admire in others:

1.

2.

3.

4.

Personality traits I dislike in others:

1.

2.

3.

4.

My good points are:

1.

2.

3.

4.

Points I could improve are:

1.

2.

3.

4.

Figure 5-5

AMERICAN ACADEMY OF PEDIATRICS
HOMOSEXUALITY AND ADOLESCENCE

In 1974, the American Psychiatric Association ended its classification of homosexuality as a mental disorder, labeling it rather as an alternate choice of sexual expression. This decision was based on the beliefs of the majority that there were insufficient data to label such individuals as being ill and that the deleterious social consequences of the pathologic designation were so grievous as to demand the declassification.

Although theories regarding the etiology of homosexuality have been based on genetic, hormonal, psychological, and environmental models, there is little reason to believe that any one of the arguments alone explains all homosexual orientation or behavior. Homosexuality has existed in most societies for as long as recorded descriptions of sexual beliefs and practices have been available. Although little agreement exists concerning the etiology of homosexuality, and any definition of terms will be arbitrary, some operational definitions are necessary.

Four assertions can be made regarding homosexuality during the teenage years:

1. Some homosexual experimental behavior is experienced by many adolescents. This may include fondling of the body or genitalia or mutual masturbation. In the vast majority of cases these homosexual encounters do not predispose to later obligatory homosexuality, but appear to be a common exploratory behavior en route to conventional heterosexual development.

2. Homosexual characteristics appear to be established before adolescence. Although many individuals do not participate in overt homosexual play during childhood, the self-conscious psychological state probably often exists before adolescence.

3. Some previously heterosexually oriented adolescents will become involved in homosexual activities if circumstances reinforce this behavior or if heterosexual alternatives are not available. This is termed facultative homosexuality. The majority of these individuals will ultimately revert to heterosexual practices when circumstances change. This situation is faced by large numbers of incarcerated teenagers, and to a lesser degree by teenagers in isosexual boarding school settings and military barracks.

4. The vast majority of behaviors should not be characterized as "male" or "female" since most are common to all young people.

Teenagers, their parents, and the community organizations with which they interact may look to the pediatrician for clarification of the medical and social issues involved when the question or fact of adolescent homosexual practices arise. An appropriate history of sexual orientation and practices must be obtained before adequate medical care can be given. The pediatrician must be entirely nonjudgmental in posing sexual questions if he or she is to be at all effective in encouraging the teenager to share his or her concerns, experiences, and beliefs.

Figure 5-5 (Continued)

Only with adequate information of this kind can there be proper medical assessment of the potential consequences of homosexual practice or fears. If the history includes open-ended questions about homosexual beliefs, practices, and experiences, then the pediatrician may elicit items that require either further investigation and evaluation, or possibly referral. If the pediatrician, on the other hand, finds it impossible to be so objective and nonjudgmental, perhaps because of religious or moral convictions about the acts involved, he or she must be honest with the patient and , after expressing personal views in a helpful and understanding manner, offer the option of referral to another professional for treatment or counseling.

The medical consequences of homosexual activity are those that primarily result from the sexual practices of fellatio, cunnilingus, and anal intercourse. Although these practices are also utilized by heterosexuals, these behaviors should always be considered when caring for the homosexual adolescent patient. Sampling sites for sexually transmitted pathogens such as Neisseria gonorrhoeae and enteric organisms should always include the pharynx and rectum in teenagers engaging in these practices. The increased incidence of hepatitis B and Giardia lamblia infestations in these individuals must be remembered as well, as should the important new epidemic of "AIDS" (acquired immune deficiency) disease expressed by lymphadenopathy, infection with unusual pathogens, or Kaposi's sarcoma.

The social consequences of homosexual orientation in an adolescent include potential difficulties in peer group acceptance, family rejection, school and institutional harassment, limited employment opportunities, legal difficulties, and social isolation. Although homosexual orientation does not appear to predispose to mental illness, the social consequences of this lifestyle in a teenager may create serious secondary emotional problems.

The American Academy of Pediatrics recognizes the physician's responsibility to provide health care for homosexual adolescents and guidance for those young people struggling with problems of sexual expression. The pediatrician can play a role in the evaluation and care of those adolescents who are concerned about their expression of sexual preference by offering reassurance to those in discomfort because of early adolescent homosexual experience; willingness to help or refer for help those in difficulty with family, peers, or institutions; and by being familiar with community resources for teenaged homosexuals and their parents if referral for social and emotional stress is indicated.

Committee on Adolescence, 1982–1983
William A. Long, Jr., MD, Chairman

CHAPTER 6

HEALTH EDUCATION

Chapter 6

HEALTH EDUCATION

A good teacher is one who becomes progressively less necessary.

—*Thomas J. Carruthers*

Unlike illness care, which intervenes with specific health problems, preventive health is an ongoing process. The cornerstone of making wellness a lifetime commitment is self-responsibility. Thus, health education relies on enhancing self-responsibility for its effectiveness.

Health education in this chapter refers primarily to curriculum-based classroom instruction that deals with healthful living habits and disease prevention. The stimulus for requiring health instruction in most states came in the wake of World War II when a large portion of recruits were found to be physically unfit to serve in the armed forces. This was considered a national disgrace requiring immediate and comprehensive action through the schools.

Today, many of the problems discussed in Chapter 4 have provided further impetus to expand the concept of health education beyond physical health and disease to include mental health issues. We now acknowledge that the major health problems are largely preventable and attributable to behaviors acquired in youth. We have learned that teaching facts does not necessarily change behavior. The thrust has shifted from preaching to *decision making*. We want young people to understand that personal health is their responsibility and that they are (or should be) in control of most aspects of their lives. Immunization against polio has almost eliminated it, but we can't immunize against teen pregnancy, drug abuse, or STDs. Success with these problems depends on education. We still must convey the facts regarding disease processes, but we must single out and emphasize those diseases that result from unhealthful living, and are thus preventable. The goal is to preempt bad habits when possible (primary prevention) and reverse them if present (secondary prevention). Tobacco use is a prime example.

It is not difficult to see that we are dealing with issues very different from other areas of learning such as mathematics and language arts. Affective skills take on central importance in dealing with health-related behaviors. For instance, the decision of a junior high student to smoke is probably related more to dealing with peer pressure than with understanding the dangers and risks of smoking.

The current framework for effective health education focuses not only on knowledge but on attitudes and skills—a shift from *health instruction* to *health promotion*. The logic of this approach is obvious when we acknowledge that health behaviors are affected by complex, often conflicting, forces. We conclude, then, that health is an applied discipline with practice of skills required.

The following definitions from the Joint Committee on Health Education Terminology (1991) delineate currently accepted usage:

Comprehensive School Health Program—A comprehensive school health program is an organized set of policies, procedures, and activities designed to protect and promote the health and well-being of students and includes health services, healthful school environment, and school health education. It should also include guidance and counseling, physical education, food service, social work, psychological services, and employee health promotion.

School Health Education—One component of the comprehensive school health program which includes the development, delivery, and evaluation of a planned instructional program for students pre-school through grade 12 and is designed to positively influence health knowledge, attitudes, and skills.

School Health Educator—A school health educator is a practitioner who is professionally prepared in the field of school health education, meets state teaching requirements, and demonstrates competence in the development, delivery, and evaluation of curricula for students and adults in the school setting that enhance health knowledge, attitudes, and problem-solving skills.

THE CLASSROOM AND THE CURRICULUM

Poor teaching in any field can be harmful to students, but incompetent health teaching can actually be injurious. When health is an orphan, taught sporadically by an uninterested or ill-prepared teacher, students develop a dislike for it. Conversely, when adequately prepared teachers (at least a college level minor in health) assume the classroom responsibility, health education can become a meaningful, even stimulating, course.

Goals of Health Instruction

The goals of health instruction are to instill in students

- resolve to attain a high level of wellness
- pride in good health

- self-responsibility for health behaviors
- application of reasoning to health problems
- use of established health principles in decision making
- consideration for the health of others
- cooperation with community health efforts

Health teaching should grow out of recognized interests and needs of students. Some phases of health teaching may best be handled by incidental instruction—problems that are of deep personal concern to a particular student. You should invite such referrals from health educators.

It is always desirable that school subjects reinforce one another. The health instructor may use math by graphing the blood pressure of students. The math teacher can use health data to demonstrate the construction of tables and charts. This type of correlation and reinforcement should always be encouraged.

Thus, we have three basic types of health instruction:

1. Planned direct instruction
2. Incidental instruction
3. Correlated instruction (cross-subject reinforcement)

Characteristics of Successful Curricula

With regard to successful health curricula, Seffrin (1992) outlines the following common elements:

- Sequentially developed (each year builds on the previous one)
- Opportunities for students to understand health in its larger social context
- Careful coordination with other subjects
- In-service programs to prepare teachers
- Outreach activities that are designed to involve parents
- Taught in the context of a healthful environment (so that health messages are reinforced rather than negated)
- Involvement of community agencies

When any of these characteristics is missing, the likelihood of success of health instruction is diminished.

Content Areas

The National Professional School Health Education Organizations recommend a core body of knowledge by major areas:

- Personal Health
- Nutrition
- Growth and Development
- Safety and Accident Prevention
- Family Life
- Prevention and Control of Disease
- Substance Abuse
- Consumer Health
- Community Health
- Environmental health

These content areas are infinitely broad, but, when focused on the ages, interests, and needs of local students, they can result in a tailor-made curriculum.

Several studies have shown a positive correlation between healthy student attitudes and the number of hours spent in health education class. Certainly, without accurate information, the likelihood of good health decisions is minimal.

Elementary vs. Secondary

A well-planned sequence of instruction progresses from personal health in the elementary grades, through a peer-group and schoolwide focus in junior high, to communitywide and national health issues in high school.

While elementary students may accept a "what" answer, secondary students want to know "how and why." Further, the desire for emancipation from adult domination in high school students lends itself to independent projects and study that enhance the ultimate goal of self-responsibility.

At the junior high level, group loyalty is important and the teacher should capitalize on the strong desire for peer approval. The differences between the sexes in junior high present instructional challenges. Physiologically and socially, 12-year-old girls are almost two years ahead of boys. Finding common interests can be problematic and may require gender specific projects for both mental and physical health learning experiences. Girls may want to learn about interpersonal relations with the opposite sex while boys are still absorbed in collecting baseball cards.

Curriculum Examples

"Core Health Education Curriculum," Figure 6-1, located at the end of this chapter, illustrates one example of specific health topics for grades 4–6. Each successive grade builds on knowledge from the preceding year. Fleshing out the topic of tobacco use and dividing objectives into knowledge, attitudes and skills results in a document similar to that shown in Figure 6-2, "Instructional Concepts on Tobacco Use." Note how the concepts are extended to the secondary level.

There are numerous excellent health curricula, but the key to successful health education is local relevance. Teachers, nurses, and others must use the curriculum in a meaningful way for their particular group of students. Lock-step state or local health curriculum requirements are anathema unless they allow expansion and contraction of specific topics or units to meet local needs. Students must first be offered what they want to know. Capitalizing on that interest gains attention and develops rapport. Later they will be more receptive to being taught what educators think they need to know.

Passive techniques are the least effective. If health instruction consists only of lectures and "canned" reading assignments, attention and interest will flag. Too many health education courses still operate in this mode. Role playing about decisions is an effective way of involving students because they must make personal decisions regarding every health topic.

You can bring a topic to life by presenting a case history to a health education class. You can also speak with authority regarding treatment of specific problems and the consequences of no treatment. The school psychologist is another valuable resource in the classroom when mental health problems are discussed.

The real challenge is linking the classroom to reality. Good grades on quizzes are nice, but seeing behaviors and attitudes change is the real goal and reward.

Textbooks

While high quality health texts abound, they should never be the controlling force in the classroom. Select and use textbook sections or chapters only as they relate to the curriculum objectives. They are a good source of background information to introduce a subject as well as suggested activities for determining attitudes and practicing skills. Using the textbook exclusively doesn't promote effective learning.

THE SCHOOL NURSE IN THE CLASSROOM

Taking the Initiative

Most health educators welcome suggestions from the school nurse regarding teaching materials, guest speakers and field trips, but they may not initiate the contact. When this is the case, you should take the initiative. A three-step process usually works well. The first step is a formal letter from the coordinator of school nurses to health educators, which officially establishes the nurse's availability in a consulting role. Figure 6-3 gives an example.

Step 2 can be a short memo from the building nurse to the local health educator suggesting a student need that should be addressed. This memo should confirm the nurse's availability to participate in classroom activities. See Figure 6-4 for a sample.

The third step is face-to-face contact to follow up your written offer and to determine the focus for a specific project. A good ice breaker for your first appearance in the classroom is to explain the school health services available to students. Opening the door and extending an invitation will almost always stimulate important student self-referrals. At the same time, you are informing the health educator and laying the ground work for future joint activities. (There are not nearly enough student referrals from health educators to nurses.) The personal problems of students cannot be dealt with in the classroom; consequently, the teacher should be sensitive to picking up on individual student needs.

Content Expert

As a content expert, you can be most helpful during question-and-answer periods, particularly with regard to current community health practices. You are also the resident expert regarding medications, both prescription and over-the-counter, and other treatment modalities. In addition you can offer, or quickly obtain, information on guest speakers—on cutting-edge topics such as organ transplants, ethics, and other topics.

Infusing Reality

You can help the classroom teacher bring credibility and specificity to health education topics. You link the classroom with the real world by translating abstract concepts into real examples and experiences. This, in turn, leads students toward becoming better consumers of health care.

Cultural Competence

Health behaviors are heavily influenced by cultural values, morals, and perceptions. Any individual wishing to enhance the effectiveness of health instruction must increase her or his awareness of the different cultures and how they impact health and education. Strategies for one culture are not necessarily appropriate or effective for another culture.

HEALTH MESSAGES OUTSIDE THE CLASSROOM

Media

A significant part of effective health education is counteracting the wrong messages that bombard children daily from the media and their environment. The first front of this battle is the school environment. If the entire school is not smoke free, then classroom attempts to prevent tobacco use will be hindered if not stopped dead in the water. Conversely, if the school lunch room has a salad bar, and offers healthy choices, students have an opportunity to practice the nutrition skills they learned in the classroom.

Media messages, particularly television and billboard advertising, send a continuous flow of negative health messages. While it is a positive step that cigarette ads have been removed from television, those for alcoholic beverages have not. Beer advertisements with strong role models are powerful influences and difficult to counteract. While adults can mentally filter ad messages, young people are like computer data banks, storing information for future retrieval and use in emulation of unhealthy behaviors.

A new children's magazine, *Zillions,* contains consumer reports for youngsters (ages 8–14). One issue reported on the TV commercials voted most misleading by young people. The overall tone develops a healthy skepticism toward advertising and brand loyalty. It is an excellent classroom teaching aid. Your school or public library probably subscribes to it.

Peers

Peers are, of course, the notorious primary source of the most "believable" information, especially when it comes to sex and drugs: "My best friend would not lie to me." No, but his facts may be all wet. For this reason, peer tutoring and mentoring is a powerful tool in health education. If seniors think it's uncool to get drunk and lose control, then tenth graders will too. Peer role models are more effective than adult role models. Kids think, "I'll be like that teacher when I'm as old as that teacher, but for now. . . ."

One caution: Older students need orientation and coaching to be good peer tutors; they can't just be turned loose with younger students.

Family

Parents and older siblings are strong determinants of health attitudes in children. They have exerted their influence for four to five years before a child begins school. When the role modeling has been good, it's easy to build on healthy behaviors. When modeling has been negative, it's an uphill struggle. Children can also have a positive effect on their families. Involving parents in determining curriculum elements and implementing health instruction is critical.

In a recent Gallup survey (1994), parents were more supportive of health instruction than school administrators. Capitalizing on this interest, you can encourage parents to effectively reinforce positive health behaviors, or at least not negate classroom messages. PTA and ad hoc advisory groups of parents are a good start. Health fairs are also a way to bring parents, students, teachers, and community health professionals together to achieve a common focus.

Health Care Community

A health education curriculum can be enhanced by integrating programming with the community. The American Academy of Pediatrics suggests five ways.

1. Bring community resources into the classroom (physicians, community nurses, dentists, and others).
2. Take the classroom into the community via field trips.
3. Send students into the community to participate in health service projects.
4. Engage community health agencies in joint planing of events. (There are a number of national health observances, such as American Heart month.)
5. Initiate a school-community interagency network to help prioritize approaches to health education in the school.

Particularly effective is a coalition of agencies and individuals formed to address such critical issues as preventing the spread of HIV in adolescents, teen pregnancy, and violence. None of these problems will be solved by schools alone.

CONVERTING FACTS TO HEALTHY BEHAVIOR

Students can achieve high test scores in health class, yet not change their attitudes or behavior. In other words, health education cannot be a self-contained classroom entity if it is to be effective. Flip back a few pages and review the section, "Characteristics of Succesful Curricula." The sixth item is: "taught in the context of a healthful environment." This includes schoolwide, community, family, and peers. Mixed messages must be minimized and the right messages must be reinforced—repeatedly. The support of administrators and parents is relatively easy to muster. Communitywide involvement and support is somewhat more of a challenge. While community agencies are a good source of materials (American Heart Association, Cancer Society, etc.), they usually have a very narrow, even organ-specific focus. You want to emphasize the concept of *comprehensive* health education.

Although health education generally refers to the curricular offering, much health education can and should take place outside the classroom. The mission in health education, in its broadest sense, is to get students to see the big picture—the social context of health. Fragmented approaches will not get the job done.

What you may refer to as *health counseling* is a one-on-one exchange with a student who has an existing or potential health problem, but every student contact is an opportunity for health education. For example, in the course of performing hearing screening on elementary students, you can stress the ill effects of loud noise on hearing. Music from cassette and CD players (particularly those with head sets) is a prime offender, as are rock concerts. Some tasks warrant protection from excessively loud chronic noise, such as use of various tools in woodshop.

You and health educators can reinforce each other's effectiveness by becoming acquainted with both roles. It requires extra effort to make health instruction and health services complementary in the school setting, but without this effort, our youth will receive less than they deserve.

ADDITIONAL NURSE ACTIVITIES

I have previously suggested that you serve on curriculum planning and textbook selection committees. These are more specialized and merit further mention because they do not fall within the usual expertise of most school nurses.

Curriculum vs. Approach

The plethora of good health education textbooks and curricular offerings can be used as valuable resources, but few packaged offerings should be used *in toto*. These materials require thoughtful application and additional activities to meet the needs of local student groups.

To focus on local needs, go back to the needs assessment you developed in Chapter 1. What are the prevalent causes of death, disease, and accidents in your community? Make sure your selection of topics or units includes these. Classroom time is at a premium. A school cannot afford to waste it on topics of little importance to the community. If health education doesn't play a role in addressing, and reducing these problems, it is not doing its job. Be focused!

Any curriculum—even one that is formally adopted and required—should be a framework to which you add your own sound judgment.

Student-directed activities are more meaningful, and students will remember them longer. Offering choices is essential. Allow students more than one way to achieve an educational objective. Good students who require little structure can do much on their own. Science projects, when well supervised, are an effective tool for discovery. Facts discovered by students stay with them—long after test scores are recorded.

When you sit on a curriculum committee, you must keep in mind the needs and interests of the local children. Packaged products do not do this; however, selected "units" may be usable as is. A good curriculum addresses all local student health problems and potential problems. It must also address an often heterogeneous group of students. Special student populations requiring consideration are those who

- are culturally or linguistically different
- have handicaps
- have academic difficulty
- are from migrant families
- are gifted and talented

Despite their differences, these students have a common need for alternate approaches to instruction in the classroom because regular classroom teaching strategies are generally inadequate for them.

A major goal of any education program is to provide all students with opportunities to advance to the full extent of their abilities. Instruction for students with special needs includes the same essential elements as instruction for general education students, but special program personnel and regular instructional personnel are jointly responsible for the modified delivery of instruction.

Textbook Committees

When the core curricular elements are in place, the next decision is whether to adopt a textbook. If the decision is yes, use the following guidelines when you serve on a textbook selection committee. A good textbook should have these characteristics:

- primary emphasis on normal well-being
- content directed to the interests and needs of students
- emphasis on mental health issues
- community health
- minimal anatomy and physiology
- age appropriate content and reading level
- numerous examples to illustrate abstract concepts
- a variety of hands-on activities
- meaningful illustrations
- suggestions for evaluation of student knowledge, attitudes, and skills

Whether a textbook is selected or not, instructional strategies should be determined. While these activities must be interest holding, they should meet specific educational objectives and not merely be fun for fun's sake. Figure 6-5 lists 91 elementary instructional activities to use for almost any topic.

Many of these can also be used at the secondary level. Some of them require careful student orientation prior to participation and a focused debriefing following the experience (city council meeting or a museum visit).

A specific example is the advertisement review in Figure 6-6, "Buy and Try." Elementary students are at the stage where they believe most of what's in print, so a review of advertisements can be eye opening. Since youngsters like to eat and food ads are plentiful, this is a stimulating way to kick off a unit on nutrition. Have students complete the "Buy and Try" worksheet on a food advertisement they have selected, then debrief two or three in class. Help them understand that manufacturers want us to buy their products (so they can profit) and may stretch or misrepresent the truth. Critical evaluation of advertising is a valuable consumer skill.

After students have completed this exercise, give them the "Advertising Techniques" fact sheet in Figure 6-7. Let them discover what they have overlooked. They will remember it far longer than if a teacher simply tells them.

The message in these examples is that the lecture is dead and textbooks are less important. Active participation is where it's at!

Sex Education

You are the content expert to ensure that instruction in human sexuality is relevant to the targeted students. You know what the problems and questions of young people are—dealing frequently with teen pregnancy, STD, and requests for contraceptive information. You can ensure that medical information represents current practice in the community and that referral resources are included. Arranging a visit to a hospital nursery brings home the round-the-clock responsibilities of parenthood. Such visits often spawn questions and stimulate thought.

Characteristics of successful sex education curricula include

- specific behavioral goals
- proven approaches
- accurate information about risks
- age-appropriate activities
- modeling and practice of communication skills
- accepted community norms
- trained staff

View of a Health Educator

Nationally involved health education specialist, Phyllis Simpson, Ph.D. (best known for her work in HIV education) outlines her view of the school nurse's role in health education:

1. Advocacy—Support the concept of comprehensive (expanded) school health education programs.
2. Role Model—Work to maintain personal health and wellness and encourage faculty wellness programs.

3. Anticipatory Guidance and Prevention—Develop strategies for one-on-one health education that are skills oriented (not primarily knowledge based).

4. Classroom Resource—Plan with the health education teacher to provide content-related presentations on leading causes of adolescent morbidity.

5. Classroom Assistance—Work collaboratively with the health education teacher to develop a skills program that is effective in delaying or preventing unhealthy risk taking.

In addition, Dr. Simpson believes that the school nurse must have a rudimentary understanding of pedagogy: social and behavioral learning theory, research in health instruction, and trends in comprehensive school health.

This view meshes nicely with the position statement from the National Association of School Nurses, which says, in part: ". . . the school nurse should use her professional preparation as a health consultant to the teacher in the classroom and as a member of the curriculum planning committee."

Finding the Time

School nurses are busy people. They have their hands full with clinic traffic and other responsibilities. How to find time to go into the classroom?

One answer is the clinic assistant or nurse aide. Having a second pair of hands to assist with clerical tasks, first aid, and routine screening frees you for more professional activities. (See the section, "School Personnel," in Chapter 9.)

Another possibility that has worked well in some schools is to have specified clinic hours. That is, have the clinic closed to nonemergency visits for one to two hours per day. Teachers and students learn the schedule quickly, making more efficient use of nurse time.

Additionally, you should look at all activities that are not direct student care to see which can be eliminated (committee meetings, paperwork, etc.).

Finally, it is reasonable to assume that computerization will streamline much of the necessary recording and reporting in the future (see Chapter 14).

When asked how school nurses can find time for classroom teaching, Sunny Thomas Alcorn, School Health Coordinator for the Texas Education Agency says, "When the school nurse comes to realize how effective she can be in the classroom as a health teacher, and how big the payoff can be, she will make time."

MAKING COMPREHENSIVE HEALTH EDUCATION HAPPEN

Comprehensive health education encompasses several concepts dealt with in this chapter:

- multidisciplinary involvement
- shift from health instruction to health promotion

- focus on mental health and social context of behavior
- schoolwide and communitywide approach
- primary emphasis on self-responsibility and decision making
- parent inclusion
- correlation and reinforcement among classroom subjects
- provision for evaluation and fine tuning.

Allensworth (1994) provides a framework for connecting the various components. See Figure 6-8. This matrix for comprehensive health education is an uncomplicated way for a school to begin to link the interrelated parts of health promotion. Sample entries are shown in the Health Services portion to guide you in the types of entries that should go in the empty boxes. The completed matrix for a given school will provide a strategy and game plan for implementing a focused health promotion program.

SUMMARY

Health education is education in the art of living. The curriculum should focus on the total person by addressing important mental health issues in addition to physical health. The cornerstone of effective health education is self-responsibility, which in turn depends on informed decision making. Unlike mathematics, biology, and language arts, dealing with attitudes and beliefs is an integral part of effective health education. The real challenge is linking the classroom to reality; good grades on quizzes are nice, but seeing behaviors and attitudes change is the goal. Through your activities in and outside the classroom, you can help forge this link with the real world and alter the current trend of risk-taking behavior, poor health, academic failure, and dropping out.

REFERENCES

1. Allensworth, D. Morbidity and Mortality Weekly Report, 41: 747–749.

2. Albrecht, Laura. "What School Children Aren't Learning About Health." *Texas Medicine* 90(6):22–23, 1994.

3. Blake, Jeanne. *Risky Times.* New York: Workman Publishing, 1990.

4. Gordon, Sol. "Family Life Education for the Handicapped." *Journal of School Health* (May 1980): 272–274.

5. Jackson, Shirley. "Comprehensive School Health Education Programs: Innovative Practices and Issues in Standard Setting." *Journal of School Health* 64(5):177–179, 1994.

6. Jampolsky, G. *Advice to Doctors and Other Big People.* Berkeley, CA: Celestial Arts, 1991.

7. Lewis, Frances. "The Evaluation of Health Education Programs for Youth." In *Principles and Practices of Student Health,* pp. 228–243. Oakland, CA: Third Party Publishing, 1992.

8. Merki, Mary. *Health: A Guide to Wellness.* Mission Hills, CA: Glencoe Publishing, 1987 (High school text).

9. Nader, P. R. "School Health Education." In *School Health: Policy and Practice*, pp. 98–109. Elk Grove Village, IL: American Academy of Pediatrics, 1993.

10. National Professional School Health Education Organizations. "Comprehensive School Health Education." *Journal of School Health* 54(8):312–315, 1984.

11. Olsen, L. *Being Healthy.* Orlando, FL: Harcourt Brace, 1990 (Grades 4–6).

12. Proctor, Susan. *School Nursing Practice* (Standard 8, Health Education), pp. 47–50. Scarborough, ME: National Association of School Nurses, 1993.

13. Roper, William. "Kids, Health, and the Media." *Journal of School Health* 63(6):273–275, 1993.

14. Schwartz, J. *Will the Nurse Make Me Take Off My Underwear?* New York: Laurel Leaf Library, 1990.

15. Seddon, Tony. *Investigating Me.* New York: Derrydale Books, 1991.

16. Seffrin, J. "Why School Health Education?" In *Principles and Practices of Student Health.* Oakland, CA: Third Party Publishing, 1992, pp. 393–409.

17. Smith, David. *Controversies in Child Health.* New York: McGraw-Hill, 1991.

18. Snyder, Alicia (ed.). *Implementation Guide for the Standards of School Nursing Practice*. (Standard 5, Health Education), 1991, pp. 25–26.

19. Toner, Patricia. *Just for the Health of It!* (Unit 1: Consumer Health and Safety Activities). West Nyack, NY: The Center for Applied Research in Education, 1993.

20. U.S. Department of Health and Human Services. *Healthy People 2000: National Health Promotion and Disease Prevention Objectives.* Washington, DC, 1990.

Figure 6-1

CORE HEALTH EDUCATION CURRICULUM
(GRADES 4–6)

TOPIC	GRADE		
	4	5	6
Vision, Hearing	X		
Nutrition/Dental	X	X	
Injury Prevention	X	X	X
Disease (communicable; noncommunicable)	X	X	X
Medications	X	X	X
Mental Health	X	X	X
Alcohol/Tobacco	X	X	X
Illegal Drugs	X	X	X
Environment	X	X	X
Human Sexualities		X	X
Health Practitioners		X	X
Community Health			X

Figure 6-2

INSTRUCTIONAL CONCEPTS ON TOBACCO USE*

	Elementary	Secondary
KNOWLEDGE: Students will learn that	A drug is a chemical that changes how the body works. All forms of tobacco contain a drug called nicotine. Tobacco includes cigarettes and smokeless tobacco.	Most young persons and adults do not smoke. Tobacco use has short- and long-term physiologic, cosmetic, social, and economic consequences. Smoking cessation programs can be successful.
ATTITUDES: Students will demonstrate	A personal commitment not to use tobacco. Pride about not using tobacco.	Responsibility for personal health. Confidence in personal ability to resist tobacco use. Support for others' decision not to use tobacco.
SKILLS: Students will be able to	Communicate knowledge and personal attitudes about tobacco use. Encourage other persons not to use tobacco.	Support persons who are trying to stop using tobacco. Identify and counter strategies used in tobacco ads. Initiate school action to support a smoke-free environment.

*Centers for Disease Control, 1994 (abbreviated).

Figure 6-3

LETTER TO HEALTH EDUCATORS FROM SCHOOL NURSE COORDINATOR

Dear Health Educator:

We often give lip service to cooperation between health education and health services. I would like to put the concept into action by making a few specific suggestions regarding the availability of school nurses to assist you in the classroom.

School nurses can be valuable resource persons and content experts in the following areas:

- growth and development
- human sexuality
- communicable and noncommunicable disease
- health maintenance / disease prevention
- ethics of health care
- health careers
- health quackery
- medication
- many others

Our nurses can obtain or serve as guest speakers, suggest field trips, serve on curriculum and textbook selection committees, and help locate free teaching materials and aids.

I hope you will call on your local school nurse to assist in one or more of these areas.

Sincerely,

Jane Doe, RN.
Coordinator, School Nurses

Figure 6-4

LETTER FROM SCHOOL NURSE
TO HEALTH EDUCATOR

Dear Health Educator (use name):

Over the last few weeks, I have seen a number of students with _____ in the school clinic. Would you be able to address this issue in your classes? I am available to join you in the classroom for such a session or to suggest materials.

Please let me know how I can help.

Sincerely,

Mary Smith, RN
School Nurse

Figure 6-5

ELEMENTARY INSTRUCTIONAL ACTIVITIES

1. advertisement review
2. art gallery
3. attitude scales
4. book cover
5. brainstorming
6. bulletin board
7. buzz groups
8. cartoons
9. case study
10. chart
11. checklist
12. city council meeting
13. collage
14. computer games
15. computer problems
16. computer reviews
17. construction
18. costume
19. creative writing
20. crosscut diagram
21. debate
22. demonstration of a technique
23. diagrams/drawings
24. diorama
25. discussions
26. editorial/essay
27. exhibits
28. experiment
29. fact file
30. fairy tale
31. field trips
32. films
33. flannel boards
34. flip book
35. game board
36. geometric shapes
37. glossary/vocabulary
38. greeting card
39. guest speaker
40. illustrated story
41. interrupted video
42. interview
43. jigsaw puzzle
44. journal/diary
45. laboratory experiences
46. letter to the editor
47. magazines
48. maps
49. minicenters
50. mobiles/models
51. movie making (video)
52. mural
53. museum
54. newscast
55. newspaper story
56. observation
57. one-act play
58. oral report
59. pamphlet
60. panel discussion
61. pantomime
62. photo essay
63. picture dictionary
64. picture with information and diagram
65. play/skit
66. poem
67. poster
68. puppet show
69. questionnaires
70. rating scales
71. rebus story
72. recordings (audiotape)
73. role playing
74. samples
75. scavenger hunt
76. science fiction story
77. score cards
78. scrapbook
79. simulation experiences
80. slides
81. songs
82. stencil
83. stitchery
84. storytelling
85. survey
86. television game show
87. town meeting
88. transparency
89. T-shirt design
90. worksheet
91. written reports

Figure 6-6

BUY AND TRY

Directions

Locate a food or beverage advertisement in a magazine or newspaper and refer to it when answering the following questions:

1. Describe the advertisement you have chosen.

2. What part of the ad caught your attention—its color, design, pictures?

3. What age group do you think this advertisement would appeal to?

4. Why do you think the company is advertising this product?

5. Have you ever tasted this food?

6. Do you believe that if you tried this food, you would think it is as good as the advertisement is trying to make it appear? Why?

7. What food product have you tried because you became interested in it while viewing its advertisement on television?

8. Was it as good as you had hoped it would be?

9. Why do you think that making all of your food choices based upon advertisements is not the most healthy thing to do?

Figure 6-7

ADVERTISING TECHNIQUES
(Food)

Attraction: Features attractive people who imply that by using the product, one can be as glamorous or good looking as they. Examples might be a stylish executive or a rugged athlete.

Having Fun: Features people enjoying themselves in activities, such as skiing, playing tennis or golf, riding bicycles, bowling, or fishing. These advertisements say that you will have fun if you eat this food.

Comparison: These advertisers say that their food choice is higher in nutrients like protein, vitamins, or minerals, for example, than that of the competition. They imply that you will be healthier if you eat what they are selling.

Status Appeal: Features exclusive settings where you find only celebrities or the very wealthy. Such advertisements suggest that if you eat the food promoted, you will be like the rich and famous.

Join the Crowd: Peer pressure is used by showing a large group having a good time. It hints that you will be included in their fun if you join them in eating a particular product.

Symbol: A symbol or a sign is used to suggest success, happiness, or some other concept. For example, a greyhound or a racehorse might exhibit speed in association with a logo. A tall tower might be used to suggest success.

Hero Endorsement: These advertisers imply that using this product will make you like the person who endorsed the product—usually a famous athlete, or a television or movie star.

Figure 6-8

MATRIX FOR COMPREHENSIVE HEALTH EDUCATION

	Schoolwide	Classroom	Health Services	Counseling
Policy			Facilitate understanding of school policies (screening, etc.).	
Environmental Change			Create supplemental learning experiences (display literature, etc.).	
Media Utilization			Publicize telephone numbers and hotlines for community agencies.	
Direct Intervention			Provide referral to community agencies as needed; organize student assistance program.	
Role Modeling and Social Support			Model support for health-impaired students.	
Instruction			Develop information exchange with teachers.	

CHAPTER 7

SPORTS ISSUES

Chapter 7

SPORTS ISSUES

===

Perhaps no where else is the mind-body synergy
more evident than in sport.

—*H. M. Chastain*

Sports have a potent influence in our culture. The emulation of the successful
athlete by youth is not ignored by advertisers, nor should it be ignored by educators. Sports participation is sometimes the first opportunity for young people
to experience an association between health theory and practice. The athletic
setting is an opportunity to teach a number of general health principles:

- personal hygiene
- first aid
- medical / dental care
- accident prevention
- nutrition
- rest and exercise

- communicable disease control
- environmental health
- emotional health
- use of leisure time
- lifetime fitness

The athletic arena should become a laboratory for demonstrating the relationships of the above components to functional living.

Working with the health educator, you can enhance your effectiveness by
capitalizing on the teachable moments to be found in sports, physical education,
and recreation. Studies of the smoking habits of students show that participation in competitive sports is an important factor in discouraging smoking.

You are most often involved in sports issues when you are called upon to interpret or obtain medical information on the potential student athlete. Should
a child participate? Are there restrictions? When should a medical reevaluation
take place? While you may not be the first-line caregiver in athletic injuries, you
will increase your effectiveness in dealing with the total child by understanding
the issues in sports health. What is the state-of-the-art treatment for a grade
III ankle sprain? What are the neurological contraindications to contact sports?
Which faulty equipment or coaching practices are likely to cause injury?

Although some athletic activities have their downside (serious injuries, undesirable psychological responses), the benefits overshadow the consequences:

- sense of accomplishment
- enhanced fitness and weight control
- experience of a commitment
- cooperation with others
- reduced stress
- development of self-discipline

In light of the decreasing physical fitness among young people, it is inappropriate to be overly critical of sports for children and adolescents. The only sport that is universally condemned by health and other organizations, including the American Academy of Pediatrics, is boxing.

BEFORE PARTICIPATION

Medical History

The primary purpose of the preparticipation examination is to screen for conditions that could predispose the athlete to injury or death. Additional functions are:

- to serve as a limited general health screening
- to evaluate physical maturation
- to detect additional risks
- to detect medical contraindications
- to identify which sports are safe for the individual
- to meet legal and insurance requirements.

The health history is the first component of the preparticipation sports assessment. The sports-related medical history has a limited scope and should focus on those conditions that are significant to athletic participation.

Determining the accuracy of information given in an athlete's history can prove difficult. False negatives are most likely to occur. For example, athletes may neglect to indicate an illness or injury that might exclude them from participation. They also may not think significant something that may, in fact, be essential to their protection or rehabilitation. Another problem may lie in discrepancies between the medical history provided by the athlete and that provided by the parent.

Figure 7-1, at the end of this chapter, illustrates a brief medical history containing the essential elements. Positive responses require further questioning to delineate specifics. If you are taking or reviewing the medical history, indicate clearly the presence of previous musculoskeletal trauma, because incompletely healed injuries predispose to more severe injuries. This allows the physician performing the physical exam to give special attention to these areas.

Many other questions may be included in the medical history; however, keep in mind that the questionnaire should be sports-specific, easily understood, and designed so that athlete, parents, and the examiner can use it easily and efficiently.

Physical Examination

The individual performing the physical examination must review the medical history carefully so that attention is focused on reported pathology. Again, the musculoskeletal system is of prime importance to the athlete. A careful assessment of the heart and blood vessels is also essential because most catastrophic events involving young athletes are related to sudden death from cardiovascular disease. The most common cardiac conditions responsible for sudden death in athletes are

- hypertrophic cardiomyopathy
- idiopathic left ventricular hypertrophy
- anomalous origin of the left coronary artery
- atherosclerotic coronary disease (familial hyperlipidemia)
- ruptured aorta

Detection of a significant heart murmur or irregular heartbeat (not suppressed by mild exercise) indicates the need for further cardiac evaluation. Thus far, sports medicine experts have not recommended including an electrocardiogram (ECG), or echocardiogram in the screening of athletes. Figure 7-2 is a standard physical exam form.

Laboratory Tests

In general, laboratory tests cause added expense with little return in the preparticipation exam. For instance, urinalysis has been a source of much anxiety because of the number of referrals it prompts due to minimal proteinuria.

Hematocrit and hemoglobin determinations are usually also unproductive. They may be normal even in athletes who are iron deficient. Tissue iron depletion is best identified with serum ferritin levels; however, this test should be reserved for athletes who have specific indications (endurance athletes or females with fatigue or diminished performance).

Maturation Staging

Assessing physical maturation is recommended to allow athletes to compete with others at similar maturity levels. The guidelines most often used are those established by Tanner. See Figure 7-3. Junior high boys benefit most from maturation indexing because of the wide range of puberty stages they demonstrate. Knowing that peak height growth velocities occur at Tanner Stage II in girls and at Tanner Stage IV in boys may aid in predicting or preventing certain injuries that occur with rapid growth.

Other Assessments

The value of additional testing is just being realized in terms of injury prevention: tests of endurance, strength, agility, body composition, and flexibility. Both reduced and excessive flexibility can predispose to musculoskeletal injury and can usually be improved considerably by a prescribed physical conditioning program. Endurance, strength, and agility can also be improved by preseason conditioning beginning at least six weeks before competition. Body composition (percent of body weight as fat) can be readily determined by calipers and serve as an objective basis for counseling in weight loss, or weight gain.

Restrictions and Contraindications

The preparticipation examination should not replace regular care by the athlete's general physician (even though many athletes and parents allow it to do so).

Clearance for participation after initial assessment should be three-tiered (Stanley 1994):

- Clearance A: unrestricted participation
- Clearance B: participation *after* further evaluation, rehabilitation, or conditioning
- Clearance C: deferred clearance due to high-risk medical condition.

An example of type C is the absence of one paired organ (eye, kidney, testicle).

Although many physicians and school districts refuse to approve participation in these cases, the courts sometimes intervene to allow the athlete to perform. After the risks have been explained to the athlete and parents, it is best to use a signed waiver as a prerequisite to participation. Figure 7-4 is an example of such a waiver.

A related issue is a request to waive all health requirements to athletic participation. These are most often made on religious grounds. Many churches have preprinted forms for this purpose. When those are not available, you can use the form illustrated in Figure 7-5.

INJURIES

Common Types

Injuries associated with sports participation most commonly affect the musculoskeletal system and fall into two categories: acute and overuse. The acute injuries receive the greatest amount of attention, as they have the greatest potential for long-term disability. Diagnosis and management of the acute injuries are relatively straightforward. Acute injuries are essentially the same, regardless of the sporting event in which they occur. Examples are ligament strains, muscle sprains, lacerations, and contusions.

The most common athletic injuries and anatomical sites are

Ligament Sprains
   ankle
   knee
   fingers/wrist

Muscle Strains
   thigh
   back
   leg
   shoulder

Contusions
   leg
   knee
   thigh

Concussions and head contusions or lacerations

Overuse
   knee
   elbow
   shoulder

Fractures
   wrist/hand/fingers

Stress Fractures
  shin (tibia)
  foot
  lower back

Fractures are actually uncommon and epiphyseal fractures are rare. The single most important indication of a fracture is the inability or unwillingness to bear weight immediately following the injury.

The ankle sprain is the most common injury in sports. Sprains of the knee, hand, wrist, and finger follow in frequency. Sprains involve stretching or tearing of ligaments around joints. The most frequent complication of this injury is recurrence—nearly always as a result of inadequate rehabilitation.

Strains involve injury to tendons and muscles ("muscle pull") and occur in sports nearly as frequently as sprains although the medical consequences are generally less severe. Strains, like sprains, are graded according to the degree of integrity remaining in the injured structure. Thus, a grade I strain is a stretched but intact musculotendinous unit. Grade II indicates partial tearing and grade III a complete rupture of the unit. Grade III strains of the musculotendinous unit are rare in young people but tendon avulsions—with an attached piece of bone—are not uncommon. The most frequent sites of muscle strains that keep athletes out of competition are strains of the hamstrings, groin, and quadriceps muscles. A frequent site of avulsion injuries is the pelvis, involving the origins of the quadriceps and, less commonly, the hamstrings.

Grade II and III strains are usually immediately disabling, may be accompanied by a "pop" or "snap," and are often quite painful. Unless an avulsed fragment is sizable, the injuries are usually treated nonsurgically. Unless the musculotendinous unit has been completely torn, rehabilitation to reestablish strength and range of motion should be started in a day or two. Lengthy periods of rest or immobilization are rarely indicated in grade I or II strains.

Overuse injuries, on the other hand, are closely related to the specific demands of the individual sports. A precise diagnosis based on the history is essential. Only then can the circumstances causing the injury be altered, thus preventing the inevitable recurrence. Examples of overuse injuries include swimmer's shoulder, tennis elbow, runner's knee, and dancer's ankle.

An entirely preventable and potentially disastrous class of injuries is the heat injuries: heat cramps, heat exhaustion, and heat stroke. These result when athletes play or practice under conditions of high heat and humidity with inadequate access to fluid and electrolyte replacement. Athletes should always have access to water, and on days when heat and humidity exceed critical levels, practices should be cancelled. Figure 7-6, the "heat index" chart, can help in making this decision.

Stress fracture in the lower back is a serious injury and is being recognized more frequently. It typically occurs during periods of rapid growth; low back pain lasting for more than two weeks suggests the need for referral to a physician familiar with this problem.

Treatment Modalities

The time-honored acronym R-I-C-E defines the treatment for most strains and sprains: rest, ice, compression, and elevation. After the first 48 hours, ice is replaced with heat. Of course, X-rays are frequently necessary to rule out a fracture, and a bone scan may be needed to rule out a stress fracture that does not show up on routine X-ray.

Other treatment modalities, such as "deep heat," (diathermy), and whirlpool have special indications. Injections of anesthetics and steroids are rarely indicated, and may be harmful.

Some injuries require surgery or specialized rehabilitation. Rehabilitation exercises are a specialized area and should be prescribed only by sports medicine physicians or knowledgeable athletic trainers.

Prevention

You may not have detailed knowledge of the pathophysiology of sports injuries, but a basic understanding will make you an effective advocate for student athletes and an ally of athletic trainers and team physicians who want to reduce injuries. A first step is understanding the amount of physical exertion and contact involved in specific sports activities. The "Classification of Sports" chart, Figure 7-7, provides an overview.

What are the causes of injuries? Grouped into general categories, they are

- poor conditioning of the athlete (lack of preseason strength and endurance training)
- poor coaching techniques (improper tackling and blocking)
- overuse (trying to get in shape too fast or performing at too strenuous a level)
- mismatched players (mixing prepubescent and pubescent junior high students)
- poor judgment by the athlete (heroic effort that exceeds strength and skill level)
- faulty equipment (proper fit of football helmets, etc.)

Probably the most important risk factor for serious knee injuries is failure to get in shape before competition in football, soccer, or volleyball.

When you see a sports-related illness or injury, ask yourself if any of these factors might be operative. If so, conferring with the coach or athletic trainer is a worthwhile proactive endeavor.

FEMALE ATHLETES

Strenuous exercise is as good for the minds and bodies of girls as it is for those of boys. The myth that competitive sports have deleterious effects on menstruation, fertility, or childbirth has no basis. Physical fitness promotes proper body function and health. In addition, competitive spirit, endurance, and durability are all traits that contribute to success in athletic activities. Until recently, such traits were generally encouraged in boys and discouraged in girls.

Although there are many physiologic and psychologic similarities between boys and girls, there also are a number of differences. The developing female skeleton is advanced about two years beyond that of the male. Puberty occurs earlier in girls than in boys. The female has a wider pelvis, which allows for better balance and performance in a sport such as gymnastics, but can create a slight body sway in running.

During exercise, a girl's body temperature rises about two degrees higher than a boy's, (girls have fewer sweat glands). Thus, female athletes build and maintain higher body temperatures during vigorous physical activity.

Until the onset of puberty, strength of boys and girls of the same age is similar. But, thereafter, boys become stronger as muscle cell growth progresses more rapidly. Girls in programs of progressive resistance weight training can substantially increase their strength, so training programs for both sexes should be essentially the same.

It is widely believed that breast injuries are common in female athletes. Consequently, female runners sometimes are urged to wear special bras. The facts do not support this view; experts do recommend, however, that female athletes with large breasts wear supportive bras made of nonelastic, sturdy, nonallergenic material.

Most injuries to young women occur during volleyball, basketball, track-and-field events, and gymnastics. They are mostly knee or ankle sprains, tendonitis, or contusions. Fractures and dislocations, especially of the elbow, have occurred in gymnastics. The severity of an injury is related to the intensity of participation. Treatment and healing of injuries is the same as for boys.

Active female athletes may experience a delay in menarche. The average age of menarche in nonathletes is 12.5 years, whereas in athletes it is 13.5 years. Physical stress, emotional stress, and excessive weight loss appear to be the most important factors. Secondary amenorrhea may occur in elite female athletes. Girls should be reminded that secondary amenorrhea is no guarantee against pregnancy; the amenorrheic athlete may start ovulating normally at any time. Contraceptive methods can be discussed with the athlete when obtaining her history. And certainly, any female athlete in whom pregnancy is a possibility should be encouraged to have a pregnancy test before continuing athletic participation.

PSYCHOLOGICAL ISSUES

Motivations and Rewards

Young people are motivated to participate in sport activities for different reasons, each carrying its own psychological impact. Numerous studies show that youngsters participate in sports primarily for fun and enjoyment. Enjoyment is defined as excitement, personal achievement, performing and improving specific skills, and comparing oneself positively with others. Fun is the feeling of happiness, and being friendly, as opposed to feeling sad and angry. Some children view being part of a team and having friends as important, and fun, whereas winning, rewards, and pleasing others are viewed as less important. The need to win is far less important to children than is often assumed by adults, although winning can be a part of the broad concept of fun.

Rewards and accomplishments are important to older youth. Teens in some studies believe that participation in sports accomplishes one or more of the following:

- develops good social skills
- enhances self-esteem
- teaches the value of cooperation
- gives people a lifelong physical activity
- develops competitive skills
- helps individuals obtain a career of status
- helps to make athletes good citizens

It seems that children and youth participate in sports to have fun and that, at a certain point in their development, they also expect some benefits and rewards to accrue from their participation in sports.

Benefits and Detriments

Studies have given evidence that participation in normal (as opposed to intense) sports activity can facilitate growth. Physical involvement is perceived to be an effective tool in the development of certain psychosocial aspects of developing youth. Such traits as character development, social adjustment, positive personality traits and attitudes, emotional control, sportsmanlike behavior, leadership skills, empathy for others, cooperation, self-discipline, self-confidence, initiative, loyalty, and self-expression have all been related to sport and its benefits.

Children who participate in sports often enjoy greater social status than do their nonparticipating peers. Some studies characterize athletes as more outgoing and socially well adjusted than nonathletes. Developmental data indicate that competitive and cooperative behaviors begin at three to four years of age and that such survival skills can be developed through normal sport experience. Evidence points to the fact that young people who participate in normal sport display both physiologic and psychological benefits. Regular physical conditioning reduces the frequency and severity of depression and thus may improve school performance. Student athletes usually have better attendance than do nonathletes.

Some problems, however, are associated with intense and stressful sport activity, and some symptoms appear under normal athletic conditions as well. For example, youth who are categorized as elite-level participants and are involved in intense competitive activity have a higher potential for burnout than those who participate on a less competitive basis. Data indicate that high and increasing numbers of children are dropping out of all types of sport involvement.

Several criticisms related to specific problems in the normal psychological development of youngsters have been leveled against competitive sports programs for young athletes. Undue pressure placed on children by overzealous adult leaders and the extreme emphasis placed by adults on winning may cause stress symptoms. When youngsters are threatened with elimination or are left out of play, they often respond with anxiety. These potential problems emphasize the need for parents and coaches to understand the psychological aspects of sport involvement and its implications for children and youth.

HEALTH PROFESSIONALS IN SPORTS

For physicians and other health care providers, the provision of services to individuals participating in sports loosely encompasses the practice of *sports medicine*. Those participating in this provider area include athletic trainers, physicians, physical therapists, nutritionists, psychologists, podiatrists, and a host of other nonlicensed personnel.

Athletic Trainers

The role of the athletic trainer includes five major areas of function:

- injury prevention
- injury care
- rehabilitation
- record keeping
- communication and education

In terms of injury prevention, the athletic trainer should be an advisor on basic conditioning programs and on the use of exercise equipment. He or she, in conjunction with the coach and equipment manager, is also responsible for making sure that playing conditions and equipment are safe prior to participation.

The athletic trainer's primary responsibility is to prevent injury, but when injuries occur, it is important that proper first aid, referral, and transportation be carried out. Injuries occur just as often at practices as they do in game play, and the trainer is usually the key person to render initial first aid.

Once an injury occurs, the athletic trainer works closely with other members of the sports medicine team or the supervising physician to implement the prescribed rehabilitation program. Intermittent testing and reevaluation of the injured athlete provide important information for both the physician and the coach regarding readiness for return to activity.

Record-keeping responsibilities include preparticipation evaluations, injury logs, and rehabilitation progress reports and insurance forms. These functions are not only important in assisting with communication, but also imperative for insurance and liability purposes.

With regard to education and communication, the trainer should assist the physician in educating the coach, athlete, parents, and administrative personnel as to injury trends, injury potential, and prevention and care of injuries.

Team Physician

The team physician, when available, is usually an orthopedic or sports medicine specialist whose role is to supervise the athletic trainers and the care of athletic injuries, and to advise on the overall conditioning program. The physician is also responsible for performing or collecting and reviewing the data from the preparticipation physical evaluation and making the final determination for fitness for participation.

The team physician provides medical coverage for competitive events, arranges referrals to family physicians or specialists, and establishes guidelines and procedures for trainers and other personnel to respond to emergencies.

Coach

Although the coach is not, strictly speaking, a health professional, he or she is an essential member of the sports medicine team.

The coach is responsible for teaching skills, a proper game philosophy and an overall safety awareness. The "win at all cost" syndrome can be dangerous and shows little regard for the safety of the student athlete. Coaches can show their concern for safety by meeting with team members and perhaps parents to inform them of potential injuries and outlining means of prevention. Football coaches in particular should warn athletes of the potential for head and neck injuries and insist on safe blocking and tackling techniques. "Spear tackling," using the head as a battering ram, can result in serious neck injuries and should be discouraged.

The coach is also responsible for first aid in the absence of the athletic trainer or school nurse.

ATHLETES WITH DISABILITIES

You may be called upon to obtain or interpret medical information on student athletes with disabilities. These disabilities may be physical (amputees, wheelchair bound), medical (diabetes, asthma, seizures), or mental (retardation, emotional disturbance). You are often an important communication channel between community physicians and athletic personnel. You may also be asked to assess illness and the advisability of sports participation in young disabled athletes.

You may be involved in Special Olympics—the annual sports event for the mentally disabled. The largest identifiable group of participants is students with Down Syndrome. One-half of these children will have congenital cardiac lesions and about one-fourth will have atlantoaxial instability. The latter condition involves joint laxity of the first two cervical vertebra; it predisposes to cervical cord injuries from neck hyperextension and can result in quadriplegia or death. It is identified by special cervical X-rays read by an experienced radiologist. Students with atlantoaxial instability should not participate in sports with high potential for neck injury (trampoline, diving, etc.).

You should encourage the use of wrist bands that list medical conditions, medications, allergies and other essential data for Special Olympic participants.

Heat precautions are especially important to observe in students with disabilities. These students often have impaired judgment regarding their capabilities and some actually have a reduced number of sweat glands (the various syndromes of ectodermal dysplasia). Salt tablets are not recommended and may be potentially dangerous for most people.

SUMMARY

Each community is unique in the way it handles health issues in sports. Whether by invitation or self-initiated action, you should be knowledgeable about the athletic activities taking place on the school campus, including provisions for managing injuries and assessing illness. The first contact should not be an emergency call to the playing field. With a prevention orientation, you can be the catalyst for developing policies for canceling practice when weather conditions are excessively hot or cold, or when an infectious disease epidemic is imminent. As with other nurse activities, making yourself available is the important first step.

GLOSSARY

Abduction	The act of drawing a limb away from the midline. (see *adduction*).
Acclimatization	Body's adaption to a new environment, especially temperature, humidity and altitude.
Adduction	The act of drawing a limb toward the midline.
Air splint	A precontoured, inflatable soft plastic splint.
Air pressure splint	Double-walled plastic tube that immobilizes a limb when the space between the walls is inflated.
Anabolic steroid	Testosterone, or a steroid hormone resembling testosterone, that stimulates anabolism.
Anabolism	Metabolic conversion of simple substances into complex compounds by cells (example: conversion of amino acids to protein).
Ankylosis	Restriction of joint motion from abnormal fibrous or bony overgrowth; permanent consolidation.
Athlete's heart	Healthy, efficient heart in well-conditioned athlete; apparent enlargement on X-ray may be from ventricular hypertrophy or increased distensibility; returns to prior size after cessation of training.
Calcium deposit	Abnormal calcification of soft tissue from traumatic insult, usually repeated episodes; in muscle it is referred to as *myositis ossificans*.
Delirium, posttraumatic	A posttraumatic neurological condition, displaying disturbed consciousness, agitation hallucinations, or disorientation.
Dorsiflexion	The act of drawing the toe or foot upward.
Drying out	Practice of purposeful dehydration for articificial weight control.
Ecchymosis	General extravasation of blood in soft tissues from blow producing skin discoloration.
Exostosis	Localized benign bony overgrowth.
Fracture, avulsion	Fracture in which a fragment of bone is torn away at the site of attachment of a tendon, ligament, or muscle.
Fracture, chondral	Fracture involving articular cartilage only.
Fracture, fatigue (stress fracture)	Fracture occurring after prolonged repetitive activity against firm resistance; no history of specific traumatic incident.
Fracture, pathological	Fracture occurring through an area that has been previously weakened by disease or tumor; usually occurs following minimal trauma.

Fracture, dislocation	Fracture near a joint at which dislocation has occurred.
Genu recurvatum	Hyperextensibility of knee, usually congenital; may be predisposing factor in internal derangement of knee.
Genu valgum (knock-knee)	Deformity, usually congenital, but may be secondary to trauma; knees abnormally close together while the space between ankles is increased; may be predisposing factor in development of recurrent dislocation of patella.
Heat fatigue	Transient deterioration in performance from exposure to heat, resulting in relative state of dehydration and salt depletion.
Hematoma	Pooling of extravasated blood in tissues or organs.
Hot spot	Early redness of skin from friction that leads to blister formation if preventive measures are not taken.
Hyphema	Hemorrhage into anterior chamber of eye.
Knee, internal derangement	Traumatic injury to knee in which lesions are produced in any of the internal structures (menisci, cruciate ligaments, tibial spine, articular cartilages, infrapatellar fat pad).
Knee, rotary instability	Abnormal external rotation of tibia on femur due to tear of the knee's medial capsule; characterized by the athlete's inability to change direction sharply (although ability to run forward is unimpaired).
Lace bite	Painful inflammation over dorsum of foot, usually over prominent ridge of base of first metatarsal; develops usually from abrasive irritation of tightly laced footwear.
Muscle atrophy	Wasting away of muscle tissue as the result of immobilization (cast), inactivity, loss of innervation, or nutritional disorder.
Muscle cramp	Painful involuntary contraction of skeletal muscle group; causes include salt depletion (heat cramp), fatigue, and reflex reaction to trauma.
Osteoarthritis	Degeneration of articular cartilage from congenital, traumatic, inflammatory, or aging factors.
Patella bipartite	Failure of patellar ossification centers to fuse, thus producing two parts; usually bilateral, symmetrical; usually asymptomatic.
Pes cavus (hollow foot)	Accentuated high longitudinal arch; may be congenital or result from neurological disorder causing muscular imbalance; clawing of toes and shortening of Achilles' tendon frequently present; excessive weight is placed on metatarsal heads and calluses develop in the underlying skin.

Pinched nerve syndrome (nerve contusion)	Term used to describe transient rootlike pain and other manifestations resulting from injury to the neck as in blocking and tackling a "stinger."
Postconcussion syndrome	Persistent variable symptoms of headache, tinnitus, dizziness, or confusion subsequent to a cerebral concussive incident.
Pronation	The act of rotating a hand or foot internally on its long axis (see *supination*).
Shin splits	Pain and discomfort in leg from repetitive running on hard surface with excessive use of foot flexors; diagnosis should be limited to musculotendinous inflammations, excluding fatigue fracture.
Spearing	Act of butting head into midsection or chest of opponent in football; hazardous to spearer (cervical spine injury) as well as to opponent (direct trauma).
Supination	The act of rotating a hand or foot externally on its long axis.
Synovitis, traumatic	Painful inflammation of the synovial membrane (inner lining) of a joint secondary to injury; characterized by the development of fluid within the joint (synovial effusion), sometimes mixed with blood (hemathrosis).
Tape burn	Skin rash at site of tape application due to mechanical effects or allergy.
Tetraplegia (quadriplegia)	Motor and sensory loss in all four extremities from spinal cord lesion at cervical level.
Tinnitus	The sensation of a ringing in ears from traumatic or other causes.
Trigger point	A focal point of irritation that, when stimulated, sets off a painful reaction referred to a distant area.

REFERENCES

1. Berkowitz, Kenneth. *Sports Injuries in Children*. Nutley, NJ: Hoffmann-La Roche, 1990.

2. Bernhardt, David. "Chest Pain in Active Young People." *Physicians and Sportsmedicine* 22(6):70–85, 1994.

3. Cantu, Robert (ed.). *Guidelines for the Team Physician*. Philadelphia: Lea and Febiger, 1991.

4. Cole, Andrew. "The Benefits of Deep Heat." *Physicians and Sportsmedicine* 22(2):77–88, 1994.

5. Cook, Robert. "Atlantoaxial Instability in Individuals with Down Syndrome." *Mental Retardation* (August, 1994):193–194.

6. Garrick, James. "Sports Medicine." *Pediatric Clinics of North America* (December, 1986): 1541–1550.

7. Geigle-Bentz, Frances. "Psychological Aspects of Sport." In *Pediatric and Adolescent Sport Medicine*. Philadelphia: W. B. Saunders, 1994, pp. 77–93.

8. Goldberg, Barry. "Sudden Death in Young Athletes." *New England Journal of Medicine* 329(1):55–57, 1993.

9. Griffin, Letha. "The Young Female Athlete." In *Pediatric and Adolescent Sports Medicine*. Philadelphia: W. B. Saunders, 1994, pp. 16–23.

10. Haycock, Christine. *Sports Medicine for the Athletic Female*. Oradell, NJ: Medical Economics, 1980.

11. Henrickson, Michael. "Recognizing Patterns in Chronic Limb Pain." *Contemporary Pediatrics* 11(3):33–62, 1994.

12. Hunter-Griffin, Letha (ed.). *Athletic Training and Sports Medicine*. Rosemont, IL: American Academy of Orthopedic Surgeons, 1991.

13. Nader, P. R. (ed.). "The Student Athlete." In *School Health: A Guide for Health Professionals*. Elk Grove, IL: American Academy of Pediatrics, 1993, pp. 336–351.

14. Peck, David. "Athletes with Disabilities." *Physician and Sportsmedicine* 22(4):590–92, 1994.

15. Petroff, Barbara (ed.). *A Pocket Guide to Health and Health Problems in School Physical Activities*. Kent, OH: American School Health Association, 1981.

16. Rachun, Alexius. *Standard Nomenclature of Athletic Injuries*. Chicago: American Medical Association, 1976.

17. Simons-Morton, Bruce. "Health-related Physical Education." In *Principles and Practices of Student Health*. Oakland, CA: Third Party Publishing, 1993, pp. 443–451.

18. Stanley, K. "Preparticipation Evaluation of the Young Athlete" in *Pediatric and Adolescent Sports Medicine*. Philadelphia, W. B. Saunders, 1994, pp. 24–33.

Figure 7-1

MEDICAL HISTORY

This *medical history form* must be completed *annually* by parent (or guardian) and student in order for the student to participate in athletic activities. These questions are designed to determine if the student has developed any condition that would make it hazardous to participate in an athletic event.

	YES	NO
1. Are you under a doctor's care?	_____	_____
2. During the past 12 months:		
a. Any hospitalizations or surgeries?	_____	_____
b. Any injuries requiring medical attention?	_____	_____
c. Any illness lasting more than one week?	_____	_____
3. Do you take medication regularly? (If yes, list on reverse side.)	_____	_____
4. Any allergies to medications or insect stings? (If yes, list on reverse side.)	_____	_____
5. Have you ever had a concussion or been knocked unconscious?	_____	_____
6. Ever had a convulsion or seizure?	_____	_____
7. Do you wear any removable dental appliance (bridge, plate, retainer)?	_____	_____
8. Do you wear eyeglasses or contact lenses?	_____	_____
9. Have you had a tetanus booster within the last 8 years?	_____	_____
10. Has any family member had sudden death or heart attack before age 50?	_____	_____

Figure 7-1 *(Continued)*

	YES	NO

11. Have you had any heart disease, murmur, extra beats, or high blood pressure?   _____   _____

12. Have you ever been dizzy or passed out from exercise?   _____   _____

13. Any joint injuries (fractures, sprains, strains, or dislocations?

_____ Neck   _____ Arm   _____ Thigh   _____   _____

_____ Back   _____ Hand   _____ Knee   _____   _____

_____ Shoulder   _____ Fingers   _____ Ankle   _____   _____

_____ Elbow   _____ Hip   _____   _____

14. Any organs missing (kidney, testicle, eye, etc.)?   _____   _____

15. Any chemical or substance use?   _____   _____

16. Any menstrual irregularities (females)?   _____   _____

17. Have you ever induced vomiting, or engaged in binge eating or purging?   _____   _____

18. Have you ever been disqualified from participation?   _____   _____

19. Do you know of any reason why there should be limits in participation in any sport?   _____   _____

_____   _____

Parent Signature   Student Signature

_____   _____

Date   Date

HISTORIA MEDICA

El padre y el estudiante necesitan llenar este formulario médico anualmente para que se le permita al estudiante participar en actividades atléticas. Este formulario es para determinar si el estudiante tiene alguna condición que lo ponga en peligro de participar en eventos atléticos.

	SI	NO
1. ¿Está usted bajo el cuidado de un médico?	_____	_____
2. Durante los pasados doce meses:		
¿Ha estado hospitalizado o ha tenido una operación?	_____	_____
¿Ha tenido lesiones que requirieron atención médica?	_____	_____
¿Ha tenido alguna enfermedad que haya durado más de una semana?	_____	_____
3. ¿Toma medicina regularmente? (Si así es, liste el tipo de medicina al reverso de esta página)	_____	_____
4. ¿Es alérgico a alguna medicina o picadura de insecto?	_____	_____
5. ¿Ha tenido alguna concusión o ha estado inconsciente por causa de un golpe?	_____	_____
6. ¿Ha sufrido de un ataque o convulsiones?	_____	_____
7. ¿Usa alguna parte de la dentadura que se pueda remover (puente, placa, frenos, etc.)?	_____	_____
8. ¿Usa anteojos o lentes de contactos?	_____	_____
9. ¿Le han aplicado la vacuna del tétano en los últimos 8 años?	_____	_____
10. ¿Algún miembro de la familia ha muerto repentinamente o de ataque al corazón antes de los 50 años de edad?	_____	_____
11. ¿Ha sufrido de enfermedades al corazón, murmullo, latidos adicionales o alta presión?	_____	_____
12. ¿Se ha sentido mareado o se ha desmayado durante algún ejercicio físico?	_____	_____

SI   NO

13. ¿Se ha lesionado alguna coyuntura (fractura, torcedura,
tirantez, ó dislocación)?   _____   _____

_____ El cuello   _____ El brazo   _____ El muslo

_____ La espalda   _____ La mano   _____ La rodilla

_____ El hombro   _____ Los dedos   _____ El tobillo

_____ El codo   _____ La cadera

14. ¿Le falta algún órgano (riñón, testículo, ojo, etc.)?   _____   _____

15. ¿Usa alguna substancia química?   _____   _____

16. ¿Tiene irregularidades en su menstruación (mujeres)?   _____   _____

17. ¿Alguna vez se ha provocado el vómito, tiene impulsos
frenéticos de comer, ó ha usado purgas?   _____   _____

18. ¿Ha sido descalificado en la participación de algún deporte?   _____   _____

19. ¿Hay alguna razón que limíte su participación en algún
deporte?   _____   _____

_____   _____
Firma del Padre o Tutor   Firma del Estudiante

_____   _____
Fecha   Fecha

Figure 7-2

PHYSICAL EXAMINATION

Student's Name: _____ Sex: M F Date of Birth: _____

Parent or
Guardian: _____ Family Doctor
or Clinic: _____

Weight _____ Height _____ Pulse _____ Blood Pressure _____

Legend: N = normal X = abnormal NE - not examined

General body build _____ Skin _____

Eye _____ Ear _____ Nose _____ Throat _____ Teeth _____ Neck _____

Lungs _____ Heart _____ Chest _____ Liver _____ Spleen _____ Spine _____

Abdominal masses _____

Joint Function: Neck _____ Shoulders _____ Elbows _____ Wrists _____ Hands _____

Hips _____ Knees _____ Ankles _____ Feet _____

*Neurological _____ Hernia _____ Genitalia (male only) _____

Optional at discretion of physician: HGB or Hematocrit _____ Urinalysis _____

Description of abnormal findings: _____

_____

I certify that I have examined this student and he or she may compete in supervised school athletic activities listed below with the exception those crossed out:

Baseball	Cross Country	Golf	Softball	Tennis	Volleyball
Basketball	Football	Soccer	Swimming	Track and Field	

Other: _____

Special instructions or special limitations: _____

_____

Date of Examination: _____ Printed or typed name
of Physician: _____

Physician's Address: _____ Signature of Physician: _____

*Important if the medical history is positive for concussion, seizures, loss of consciousness, or other neurological finding.

Figure 7-3

TANNER STAGES OF SEXUAL DEVELOPMENT

Boys

Stage I	Prepubertal
Stage II	Testicular enlargement (2.5 cm length)
	Scrotal thinning and increased pigment
Stage III	Increasing testicular size
	Increasing penile growth (6 cm length)
	(5 cm circumference)
	Pubic hair
Stage IV	Increasing testicular size, penile size, and amount of pubic hair
	Axillary hair
	Palpable prostate
Stage V	Testes and penis adult size
	Pubic hair triangular
	Axillary hair abundant

Girls

Stage I	Prepubertal
Stage II	Breast tissue only
Stage III	Breast tissue 2–11 cm
	Pubic hair
Stage IV	Breast tissue increasing
	Pubic hair increasing
	Axillary hair
	Menarche
Stage V	Adult breast, genitalia, and pubic hair

Figure 7-4

PAIRED ORGAN WAIVER

I, _____ , parent or legal guardian of

_____ , a student at _____

School, wish my child to participate in the [football] program.

He/she has only one [eye; kidney; testicle, etc.] and I am aware that participation in [football] could possibly result in an accidental injury that might affect the function of the good [eye, kidney, testicle, etc.].

We have consulted our doctor, who has given consent for participation.

We agree that if our son or daughter is allowed to participate in [football] and other sports activities, we will release the _____ School District, its coaches and other employees from any liability, damages, or claims resulting from any injury to the remaining [eye, kidney, testicle, etc.] that might be received while participating in such sports activities.

_____

(Parent/guardian)

_____

(Date)

Copies: Athletic Director

       School Attorney

       Director of School Health

RENUNCIA AL DERECHO DE DEMANDA LEGAL POR LA PERDIDA DE UN ORGANO ANATOMICO

Yo, _____ padre o tutor del estudiante de

la Escuela _____ , deseo que mi hijo/a participe en el programa (football).

El/ella sólo tiene un ojo, riñón, testículo, etc., y estoy de acuerdo en que su

participación en (football) podría resultar en un accidente o lesión, la cual puede afectar la

función del otro órgano anatómico (ojo, riñón, testículo, etc.).

Hemos consultado a nuestro doctor y él/ella da su consentimiento para que nuestro

hijo/hija participe en dichas actividades.

Estamos de acuerdo en renunciar a nuestro derecho de demanda legal contra el

Distrito Escolar de _____ , sus entrenadores y otros empleados, en

caso de cualquier daño que pueda surgir de una lesión recibida en el órgano en función

(ojo, riñón, testículo, etc.) durante su participación en dichas actividades deportivas.

_____

(Padre/tutor)

_____

(Fecha)

Copias: Director de Atletismo

Abogado de la Escuela

Director de la Escuela de Salud

Figure 7-5

RELIGIOUS EXEMPTION FROM HEALTH REQUIREMENTS FOR SPORTS*

I hereby affirm that

1. I am a member of the _____
    Name of church

    and

2. Requirements for physical examination and immunizations for sports conflict with the tenets and practices of my religion.

Name of student _____

Name of parent or guardian _____

Address _____ Phone _____

_____   _____
Date   Signature of parent or guardian

I am an ordained minister of the above-named church, a recognized religious organization, and have access to the membership records. The above-named person is a bona fide member of the church. Immunization, physical examinations, and other health requirements are contrary to the tenets and practices of the _____
Name of church

Name _____

Address _____ Phone _____

_____   _____
Date   Signature of church official

*This exemption does not apply in times of emergency or epidemic declared by the State Health Commissioner.

EXONERACION RELIGIOSA DE LOS REQUISITOS DE SALUD PARA DEPORTES*

Yo por medio de esto afirmo que

1. Soy miembro de la _____
   Nombre de la iglesia

2. Requisitos como exámen físico y vacunas para deportes interfieren con las creencias y prácticas de mi religión.

Nombre del estudiante_____

Nombre del padre ó tutor_____

Dirección/Teléfono _____

Fecha _____   _____
Firma del Padre ó Tutor

Yo soy el pastor de la iglesia mencionada, una organización religiosa reconocida, y tengo

acceso a los requistros de membresía. La persona mencionada es un miembro de buena

fé de la iglesia. Vacunación, exámenes físicos, y otros requisitos de salud son contrarios a

las creencias y prácticas de la _____
Nombre de la iglesia

Nombre _____

Dirección_____ Teléfono _____

Fecha _____   _____
Firma del Funcionario de la iglesia

*Esta exoneración no aplica en tiempos de emergencia ó epidemia declarados por el Comisario Estatal de Salud.

Figure 7-6

APPARENT TEMPERATURE SCALE (HEAT INDEX)*

Relative Humidity (%)

Temp *F	30%	40%	50%	60%	70%	80%	90%
86	84.4	86.3	88.3	91.0	95.0	99.4	104.6
88	86.5	88.8	91.4	94.9	99.8	<u>105.6</u>	111.8
90	88.8	91.5	94.9	99.3	<u>105.2</u>	112.3	119.5
92	91.2	94.4	98.9	104.3	111.3	119.5	127.7
94	94.0	97.6	103.3	<u>109.9</u>	118.2	127.1	136.3
96	96.9	101.2	<u>108.1</u>	116.1	125.4	135.1	145.3
98	99.8	<u>105.1</u>	113.2	122.4	132.8	143.4	154.6
100	103.0	109.3	118.6	128.9	140.4	152.0	164.2
102	<u>106.1</u>	113.8	124.3	136.0	148.3	160.9	174.1
104	109.5	118.7	130.4	143.3	156.6	170.2	184.4
106	113.4	124.0	136.9	151.0	165.3	179.9	195.1
108	117.7	129.7	143.8	159.1	174.4	190.0	206.2
110	122.4	135.8	151.1	167.6	183.9	200.5	217.7

80–94 = Very Warm: Fatigue possible with prolonged exposure and physical activity.

95–104 = Hot: Heat cramps and heat exhaustion possible with prolonged exposure and physical activity.

105–129 = Very Hot: Heat cramps or heat exhaustion likely. Heatstroke possible with prolonged exposure and physical activity.

130+   = Extremely Hot: Heatstroke imminent with prolonged exposure and physical activity.

*Adapted from Texas Department of Health, 1994. (Underlined index temperature indicates level at which sports practice cancellation should be considered.)

Figure 7-7

CLASSIFICATION OF SPORTS

Contact/ Collision	Limited Contact	Noncontact		
		Strenuous	Moderately Strenuous	Nonstrenuous
Boxing*	Baseball	Aerobic dance	Badminton	Archery
Field hockey	Basketball		Curling	Golf
Football	Diving	Discus	Table tennis	Riflery
Lacrosse	High jump	Javelin		
Martial arts	Pole vault	Shot put		
Soccer	Gymnastics	Running		
Wrestling	Ice Skating	Swimming		
	Softball	Tennis		
	Volleyball	Track		
		Weight lifting		

* Not recommended for any young person

EMPLOYEE HEALTH

Chapter 8

EMPLOYEE HEALTH
===

> Never tell people how to do things. Tell them what
> you want to achieve and they will surprise you
> with their ingenuity.
>
> —*Gen. George S. Patton*

Optimum physical and mental health of school employees is essential to an effective education program. Absent or poorly functioning employees cannot support quality learning for students. Consequently, enlightened school districts have provisions for most, or all, of the following:

- adequate health benefits
- sick leave (including maternity leave)
- wellness and health promotion programs (stress reduction, smoking cessation, etc.)
- assessment of environmental hazards (Chapter 10)
- comprehensive safety measures
- return to work with limitations (light duty; work hardening programs)
- rewards for good attendance
- early intervention for drug and alcohol abuse
- mental health assessment and treatment
- hiring and placement policies consistent with the Americans with Disabilities Act
- open communication and planning with employee and teacher unions
- consultation with school health professionals
- paid outside medical consultation
- case-by-case decision making

Local needs and constraints will dictate the extent to which each of these is provided. All should be considered carefully for their contribution to the educational mission of schools.

ILLNESS IN THE WORK SETTING

School personnel are neither healthier nor less healthy than workers in other settings. The business sector, which must show a profit to survive, has been quicker than school systems to recognize the value of strong employee health programs. The end product of education—student learning—is less easy to measure in terms of employee contribution. And, since employee health programs may not show immediate results, schools have been reluctant to make the investment at a time when numerous other demands are being made on local budgets. Such programs may not appear cost-effective over a 12-month budget cycle, but with the advent of strategic planning, the benefits have become easier to see. Large expenditures for Workers' Compensation cases have also nudged schools into taking a fresh look at employee health programs. Having provisions for immediate referral for evaluation and treatment of on-the-job injuries is a proven cost cutter.

General Health Problems

Many health problems are age related: cancer, hypertension, degenerative diseases, diabetes, and many others. Early recognition and treatment keep teachers in the classroom and other employees on the job; the lack of them interrupts the educational process.

Work-related Illness and Injury

The most common work-related incidents are slips and falls. While these have always been dealt with, they continue to occur and require constant surveillance of the environment for hazards, and safety training for prevention. The most successful efforts have come from programs that reward reduction in worker injuries—many of them financial—and modify the environment to reduce risk. Reduction in the incidence of computer-related illness is an example of the latter. Carpal tunnel syndrome can be greatly reduced with simple measures involving adjustment of chair and keyboard height to allow the wrists to function in a straight rather than a flexed position. Similarly, eye strain is reduced by having the copy at the same distance and height as the computer screen (so the eyes do not have to refocus with each glance, producing strain). Both measures can improve productivity of secretaries and data personnel who spend their days at a computer terminal.

Medical Leaves

The time-honored provision of a fixed number of "sick days" is adequate for most employees. The challenge comes in making provisions for employees with chronic, nonwork-related conditions that cause them to use their sick days early in the school year. The solution lies in better health care, which in turn can be realized through more comprehensive health benefits. An example is an employee with asthma. If this employee lacks health care benefits, and all medical expenses are out-of-pocket, the employee is less likely to receive adequate care for the asthma and will miss more work days. Universal health insurance for employees solves this problem.

Involuntary medical leave is sometimes necessary for the conscientious employee who comes to work no matter what. Without this provision, long-term productivity is negatively impacted. A high-risk pool of sick days or salary funds (contributed by employees or the school district) can ease this problem.

Returning to Work with Limitations

Physical limitations that make adequate job performance difficult or impossible pose a unique challenge. This most often arises in jobs with high physical demand. Communication with the managing physician is essential. Figures 8-1 and 8-2, at the end of this chapter, illustrate a suggested letter and form for communication with physicians regarding employee limitations.

Maternity Leave

Adequate maternity leave for uncomplicated pregnancy is a must, as are provisions for postdelivery complications. Paternal leave and leaves for adoptions are more difficult to administer fairly, but should be considered for optimal physical and mental well-being of employees.

Reducing Employee Absences

Most employees do not want to miss work and certainly don't want their pay docked; however, poor planning, or inadequate policies and health care may lead to both. All of the program elements listed at the beginning of the chapter contribute to better employee attendance.

THE EMPLOYEE ASSISTANCE MODEL

Support vs. Discipline

Until recently, only disciplinary procedures were used by most school districts to "keep employees in line." Studies from the business world have shown that a helping mode is more effective in keeping employees on the job whether the problem be alcohol abuse, undue stress, or another health issue. Support programs that restore productivity are more effective than pure disciplinary models. Such programs are referred to as *employee assistance programs* (EAP).

EAPs allow employees to present themselves and their problems to a neutral, supportive person (often an EAP coordinator) for assessment and help. This new step is interposed between flagging performance or attendance and ordinary discipline procedures as illustrated in Figure 8-3. Urban school districts will have larger EAPs, but one individual can constitute such an office or division. The EAP head can be a psychologist, counselor, nurse, social worker, or other helping professional. The primary qualification is experience with the types of problems to be handled. Out-of-district mental health professionals are also desirable for the assessment and treatment of more difficult problems, although this can sometimes be managed through the employee's individual health plan. Since most employees want to be well and do a good job, they are usually willing to sign an agreement or contract to follow the prescribed rehabilitation plan. Failure to do so causes action to revert back to disciplinary procedures and sometimes dismissal, but the employee has been given every chance for recovery.

Serious psychiatric disorders do not always respond to treatment, and dismissal may still be necessary: schizophrenia and multiple personality disorder fall in this group. Either way, a school district and its students are better off for having made the effort to assist the troubled employee; many are salvaged and returned to productivity, others who might have a negative impact on the educational process are removed.

To introduce employees to the EAP, distribute general flyers to all employees. The school can also send personalized letters to personnel returning from leave following serious chronic problems. See Figure 8-4 for a sample letter. Self-referral is first offered. At other times it may be necessary for a supervisor to make an administrative referral to the EAP. The latter action is necessitated by the employee's failure to acknowledge the problem, as may be the case with the alcoholic. Reluctance to make self-referrals is also seen in individuals who feel there is a stigma to receiving such help. In either case absolute confidentiality and sensitivity are essential.

EAP records should be kept separate from personnel files until such time as disciplinary action or dismissal is necessary. This provision will facilitate both self- and administrative referrals and promote the helping relationship.

The employee without health insurance, most often a paraprofessional, poses a particular challenge because she or he may have no primary physician or medical home; the school district must then spend consultation funds. For this reason, schools should make every effort to provide universal health coverage.

Wellness Programs

Thus far problems that are already interfering with job performance or attendance have been discussed. Ideally, EAPs should be proactive and preventive in their approach. Programs in this category are

- smoking cessation
- weight reduction
- exercise (aerobics, etc.)
- mammograms
- stress reduction
- cardiac risk screening

Making these activities available at work accomplishes three things:

1. sends a positive message about the employer
2. allows the employee to take charge of health behaviors
3. increases employee productivity through better physical and mental well-being.

Numerous studies have documented the cost-effectiveness of such programs, although it may take three years to document the overall savings to a school district. The goodwill generated will, however, produce immediate benefits.

AMERICANS WITH DISABILITIES ACT

Employees with chronic disabling conditions must be evaluated in light of the Americans with Disabilities Act (ADA). The ADA prohibits discrimination in all employment practices, including job application, hiring, firing, advancement, compensation, training, and other privileges of employment. It applies to recruitment, advertising, tenure, layoff, leave, fringe benefits, and all other employment-related activities.

Employment discrimination against "qualified individuals with disabilities" is prohibited. This includes applicants for employment and employees. The law states: "An individual is considered to have a disability if s/he has a physical or mental impairment that substantially limits one or more major life activities . . . (seeing, hearing, speaking, walking, breathing, performing manual tasks, learning, caring for oneself, and working)." Individuals with epilepsy, paralysis, HIV infection, a substantial hearing or visual impairment, mental retardation, or a specific learning disability are covered, but an individual with a minor, nonchronic condition of short duration, such as a broken limb or flu, generally would not be covered.

A "qualified" individual with a disability is a person who meets skill, experience, education, or other requirements of a position, and who can perform the "essential functions" of the position with or without "reasonable accommodation." Examples of reasonable accommodations include

- making existing facilities readily accessible to an individual with a disability

- restructuring a job
- modifying work schedules
- acquiring or modifying equipment
- providing qualified readers or interpreters
- appropriately modifying examinations, or training or other programs

An employer has no obligation to find a position for an applicant who is not qualified for the position sought, or to provide personal use items such as glasses or hearing aids.

The ADA treats the use of medical information differently at three stages:

- pre-offer of employment
- post-offer of employment (or conditioned offer of employment)
- current employment

Medical Examinations

An employer may not require a job applicant to take a medical examination before making a job offer. It cannot make any preemployment inquiry about a disability. An employer may, however, ask questions about the ability to perform specific job functions and ask an individual to demonstrate how she or he would perform these functions. An employer may condition a job offer on the satisfactory result of a post-offer medical examination if this is required of all entering employees in the same job category; for instance, an applicant for school bus driver who had poorly controlled epilepsy would not have to be placed in this position. A post-offer medical examination may disqualify an individual if the employer can demonstrate that the individual would pose a "direct threat" in the workplace—one that could not be reduced through reasonable accommodation. See Figure 8-5 for a sample policy statement.

Tests for illegal drugs are not medical examinations under the ADA, nor are individuals who chronically use illegal drugs protected under the ADA.

Reasonable Accommodations

An employer is not required to make an accommodation if it would impose an "undue hardship," which is defined as an action requiring significant difficulty or expense. Factors included in this determination include the nature and cost of the accommodation in relation to organizational size and resources, and nature and cost of the accommodation . If the cost of an accommodation would impose an undue hardship on the employer, the individual with a disability should be given the option of paying a portion of the cost.

The ADA does not override health and safety requirements established under federal laws even if a standard adversely affects the disabled individual's employment. The ADA does override state or local laws where such laws conflict with ADA requirements.

Work-related injuries do not always cause physical or mental impairment severe enough to "substantially limit" a major life activity. A laceration that heals without producing disability is one example. An employer must consider work-related injuries on a case by case basis to know if a worker is protected by the ADA. Most minor injuries are covered under Workers' Compensation.

An employer may refuse to hire or fire a person who knowingly provides a false answer to a lawful post-offer inquiry about his or her condition.

Figure 8-6 illustrates one example of a form for use as a preliminary assessment of a disabled employee who is experiencing job performance difficulties. Additional information from an outside evaluation (as from a medical or rehabilitation specialist) may be required to determine what a reasonable accommodation might be. The decision tree in Figure 8-7 can help determine whether a permanent disability exists and, if so, whether an employee can return to his or her former job and function adequately (with or without accommodations).

Mental Impairments

The following mental impairments are covered under ADA:

- retardation
- organic brain syndrome
- emotional or mental illness
- specific learning disabilities

Individuals with AIDS, and recovered drug abusers and alcoholics who have undergone treatment are also covered under the ADA.

Excluded Conditions

The ADA excludes certain conditions from the meaning of "disability":

- homosexuality or bisexuality
- sexual behavior or gender identity disorders
- compulsive gambling
- pyromania
- kleptomania
- obesity
- pregnancy
- current use of illegal drugs
- current alcoholism in individuals who cannot perform a job satisfactorily

Food service employers are not required to hire an applicant with any of these infections:

- salmonella
- shigella
- staphylococcus
- type A hepatitis
- campylobacter
- entamoeba histolytica
- pathogenic E. coli
- giardia lamblia

One possible accommodation is to offer infected individuals alternative employment that does not involve food handling.

HIV/AIDS

HIV-positive employees and those with AIDS pose unique problems. The criteria for work continuation include

1. adequate physical stamina
2. mental competency (absence of dementia)
3. absence of infectious fluid production (weeping skin lesions, nosebleeds, untreated tuberculosis, etc.)

Figure 8-8 illustrates one format for the evaluation of the HIV-positive individual.

Once completed, the form should be kept confidential and stored in a locked file in the Central School Health Services office or other appropriate place. The evaluation should be repeated every two to three months.

It should be remembered that for every known HIV-positive employee, there will be five to ten who are unknown to the school district. About half of the states have laws preventing mandatory HIV testing.

PRIVACY ISSUES

The human relations problems that arise from unrestricted access to personnel records are significant. If an employee is damaged by information being released too widely (health record, discipline history, or other matters), the employee may sue the employer for invasion of privacy or defamation.

A separate but related issue is the right of employees to have access to their own personnel records. A majority of states require that such access be provided by public employers, such as school districts.

Privacy is an extremely broad concept. An employer concerned that a particular action may involve invasion of an employee's privacy should consult an attorney.

RISK MANAGEMENT

Risk management comprises all measures to control costs related to employee injury and illness, as well as damage or theft of property. The risk management division of a school district usually administers Workers' Compensation—the program responsible for financing medical care of injured employees and pay for lost time. Risk management focuses on financial liability awareness. It is the centralization of loss control operations and the search for wall-to-wall insurance coverage for property. Employee safety is a key concern of risk management, but the primary mission is to safeguard corporate assets.

Getting injured workers back to work as soon as possible reduces cost; timely evaluation and appropriate treatment must be arranged. Although employees have a choice of treatment resources (from family physician to hospital emergency room), it is best to prearrange care with a professional or agency with experience in work-related injuries. Delay in evaluation and treatment often prolongs morbidity and impedes early return to work. Hospital emergency rooms constitute the most expensive form of care and should be reserved for the more serious or life-threatening injuries.

Core activities of a typical risk management program include

- coordinating safety programs, loss prevention, and injury claims control
- processing employee injury claims
- purchasing cost-effective property insurance
- ensuring compliance with laws and government agencies (e.g., Environmental Protection Agency)
- analyzing accident data to identify risk exposure

BLOODBORNE PATHOGENS

The Occupational Safety and Health Administration (OSHA) standard requires employers to take certain actions with respect to any employee who can "reasonably anticipate" contact with body fluids as part of the job. The standard, known as the *Bloodborne Pathogens Rule*, includes the following requirements:

- identify potential exposure risks
- implement a written infection control plan
- institute work practice controls
- regulate housekeeping, waste, and laundry
- offer hepatitis B vaccine and postexposure follow-up
- label containers of infectious materials

- institute training programs
- maintain records for employees with exposure potential.

School nurses have occupational exposure to blood and should be the beneficiaries of these protective measures. Many states are developing guidelines that track the OSHA standards.

SCHOOL NURSE ROLE

As a school nurse, you have special knowledge of health care and an understanding of the need for confidentiality and documentation. This knowledge makes you a useful resource in all areas covered in this chapter—particularly in identifying and communicating with community health personnel.

When you are first consulted regarding an individual employee health matter, be sure to create a file. It is unwise and legally naive to provide curbstone or telephone consults without creating a record. Figure 8-9 illustrates a useful form for that purpose. You can keep progress notes of further contacts or actions on the reverse side.

When an employee's attendance or performance appears adversely affected by a possible health problem, physician input is needed. Figure 8-10 is a suggested letter to the employee's physician soliciting medical input. A records release authorization signed by the employee should also be included. It is risky to rely on the employee as the only source of information, and general statements from the doctor do not always address all relevant issues. Non-health professionals located in departments of personnel, risk management, and others want medical prognoses stated with precision. You can help administrators understand that the same illness or injury in one employee may not run the same course in another employee. This uncertainty must be brokered through frequent communication between school district and managing physician. You are probably the best person to do this.

SUMMARY

Too many school districts still lack a comprehensive approach to employee health. The quality of the total educational program suffers. As longtime advocates for students, nurses can have a positive influence by expanding their advocacy to employees. See Figure 8-11, National Association of School Nurses "Resolution on Wellness Programs."

REFERENCES

1. Engelberg, A. (ed.). *Guide to the Evaluation of Permanent Impairment.* Chicago: American Medical Association, 1988.

2. Freeman, S. *Injury and Litigation Prevention.* New York: Van Nostrand, 1991.

3. Greenspan, A. (ed.). *Medical Employer's Guide.* Bedford, TX: Business Publishing, 1993.

4. Lavy, B. (ed.). *Occupational Health.* Boston: Little, Brown, 1988.

5. McCunney, R. *Handbook of Occupational Medicine.* Boston: Little, Brown, 1988.

6. Meyerson, A. (ed.). *Psychiatric Disability: Clinical, Legal and Administrative Dimensions.* Washington, DC: American Psychiatric Press, 1987.

7. Monagle, J. *Risk Management: A Guide for Health Care Professionals.* Rockville, MD: Aspen Publications, 1985.

8. *The President's Health Security Plan.* Washington, DC: The White House Domestic Policy Council, 1993.

9. U.S. Equal Employment Opportunity Commission. *The Americans with Disabilities Act: Questions and Answers.* Washington, DC, September, 1992. (1-800-669-3362)

10. Wallace, H. et al. (eds.). "Employee Health in Schools." In *Principles and Practices of Student Health,* Vol. 2, pp. 360–68. Oakland, CA: Third Party Publishing, 1992.

Figure 8-1

LETTER TO PHYSICIAN
(employee limitations)

Dear Doctor _____ :

Reference is made to our employee and your patient,_____.
Limitations were listed on the Medical Clearance form that you signed recently. We need clarification regarding the compatibility of those limitations with the physical and environmental demands of the employee's position. Enclosed is a checklist of essential physical requirements which will enable you to determine whether your patient is able to work under the conditions circled.

Please underline "is" or "is not," sign the form and return it to my office. If you have questions or prefer to communicate this information verbally, please feel free to call me at

_____ .

Sincerely,

Director, Health Services

Figure 8-2

MEDICAL EVALUATION OF LIMITATIONS

1. Employee's Name _____ Social Security No. _____

2. Position Title: _____

3. Brief description of what position requires employee to do physically:

4. Functional and environmental requirements of employee's position. (circle)
   (Completed by employee's supervisor)

A. FUNCTIONAL REQUIREMENTS

Heavy lifting/carrying (45 pounds and over)
Moderate lifting (15–44 pounds)
Light lifting (under 15 pounds)
Straight pulling (hours)
Pulling hand over hand (hours)
Pushing (hours)
Reaching above shoulder
Both hands required
Sitting (hours)
Walking (hours)
Standing (hours)
Crawling (hours)
Kneeling (hours)
Repeated bending (hours)
Climbing, legs only (hours)
Climbing, use of legs and arms
Both legs required
Operation of truck or other motor vehicle
Ability for rapid mental and muscular
coordination simultaneously
Near vision at or near 20/20
Far vision at or near 20/20
Ability to distinguish basic colors
Hearing (aid permitted)
Hearing without aid
Specific hearing requirements (specify)
Emotional/Mental Stability (specify on
reverse side)
Other (specify)

B. ENVIRONMENT

Outside (hours)
Excessive heat
Excessive cold
Excessive humidity
Excessive noise
Dust
Fumes, smoke, or gases
Slippery or uneven walking surfaces
Working around machinery with moving
parts
Working around moving objects or
vehicles
Working on ladders or scaffolding
Working below ground
Unusual fatigue factors (specify)
Working with hands in water/chemicals
Vibration
Working closely with others
Working alone
Protracted or irregular hours of work
Other (specify below)

Physician Statement: The above named
individual (is; is not) able to work under
the conditions circled above.

_____   _____
Physician Signature   Address

_____   _____
Date   Telephone

Figure 8-3

EMPLOYEE ASSISTANCE PROGRAM AND DISCIPLINARY PROCEDURES

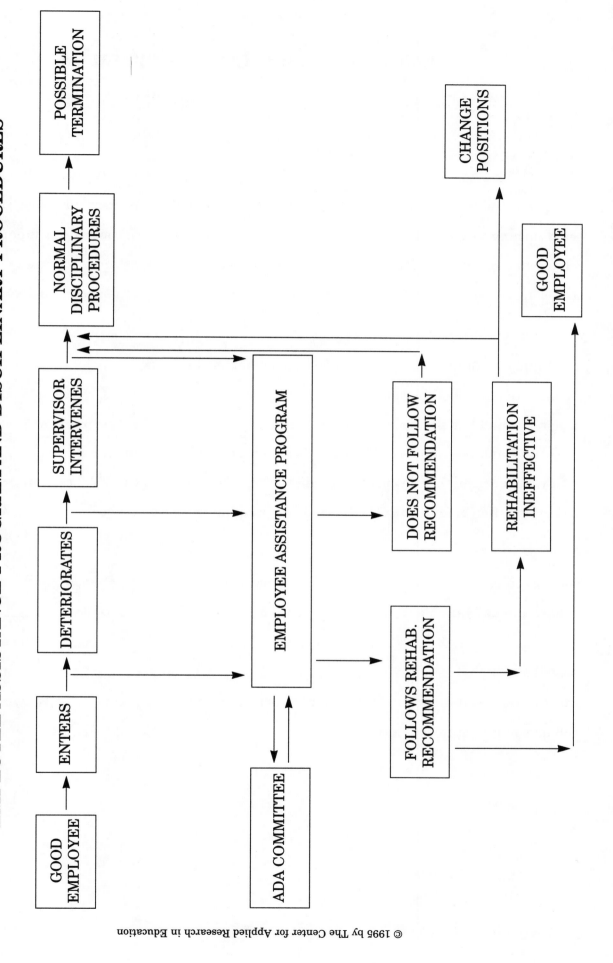

Figure 8-4

EMPLOYEE ASSISTANCE LETTER

Dear [Employee]

The _____ School District has an Employee Assistance Program to help personnel through periods of extraordinary life challenges. We recognize that employees returning to active duty following a leave of absence may have concerns or unique needs related to their work. It has been our experience that many employees returning to active status appreciate and profit from having someone they can turn to for individual support.

The Employee Assistance Program has been established to provide our personnel with a resource to meet their needs. _____ is Director of Employee Assistance and has the responsibility for drawing upon district and community resources to assist an employee who has unique needs or concerns. The Director can serve as a liaison with you, your treating physician, and district resources to assist you. All communications and information shared with the Director are maintained in confidence.

Should you or your doctor feel that return to active duty would be enhanced by the professional support available through the Employee Assistance Program, contact _____ _____ at _____ ; the office is located at _____ . Our employees are our greatest resource; it serves all parties to maintain their productivity. We wish you well as you return to active status.

Sincerely,

Personnel Director

cc: Treating Physician

Figure 8-5

SAMPLE SCHOOL DISTRICT POLICY
PHYSICAL EXAMINATIONS AND
COMMUNICABLE DISEASES

Communicable diseases include, but are not limited to, measles, influenza, viral hepatitis-B (serum hepatitis), human immunodeficiency virus (HIV infection) and AIDS, leprosy, and tuberculosis. Employees with communicable diseases, whether acute or chronic, shall be subject to the following provisions.

The information that an employee has a communicable disease shall be confirmed by one of the following methods:

1. The employee brings the information to the District's attention.

2. The employee confirms the information when asked.

3. If the Superintendent or designee has reason to believe that the employee has a communicable disease and is unable to perform the job or poses a threat to self or others, the employee may be asked to submit to a medical examination to determine whether the employee's physical condition interferes with the performance of regular duties or poses a threat to self or others.

   The results of such an examination shall be kept confidential except that the Superintendent or designee shall be informed of restrictions in duties and necessary accommodations. First aid and safety personnel may also be informed to the extent appropriate if the condition may require emergency treatment.

The Superintendent or designee shall obtain medical advice from local health authorities or private physicians on:

1. The nature of the risk, i.e., how the disease is transmitted.

2. The duration of the risk, i.e., how long the employee shall be infectious.

3. The severity of the risk, i.e., what is the potential harm to third parties.

4. The probabilities that the disease shall be transmitted and shall cause varying degrees of harm.

Figure 8-5 (Continued)

5. Whether the employee's condition interferes with the performance of regular duties. This determination shall be made by a physician who has performed a medical examination of the employee.

If the Superintendent or designee determines that work restrictions, reassignment, or exclusion may be appropriate, the Superintendent or designee shall determine whether the employee is a "disabled person." If it is determined that an employee is disabled, the Superintendent or designee shall also determine if the employee is otherwise qualified for employment. With respect to employment, a "qualified disabled person" is a handicapped person who, with reasonable accommodation, can perform the essential functions of the job in question.

If it is determined that an employee is a "qualified disabled person," the employee must be reasonably accommodated. Accommodation is not reasonable if it poses undue financial or administrative burdens or fundamental alterations in the nature of the job.

Whether an employee is disabled or not, the Superintendent or designee, based on the medical information and the requirements of the job, shall determine what exclusion or modification in job duties or assignments is appropriate, if any.

An employee may be excluded from work if the Superintendent or designee, in accordance with this policy, determines that the employee poses a risk of contagion to other employees or students, the employee poses a threat to his or her own health by remaining on the job, or the employee's physical condition interferes with the performance of regular duties.

The employee may present evidence to the Superintendent or designee of any information relevant to the employee's fitness to continue the performance of regular duties.

Employees who are excluded from work may be placed on any sick leave or temporary disability leave to which they are entitled.

Figure 8-6

ADA ON-SITE ASSESSMENT

1. Employee _____ Date _____

2. Job Title/Description (physical requirements): _____

_____

3. Site: _____

4. Evaluation: _____

   A. Diagnosis/Medical History: _____

   B. Physician prescribed limitations: _____

   C. Duration of limitations _____

   *D.   Site visit/observation _____

      1. Description of work area (furniture, equipment, etc.) _____

      2. Employee interview (description of job site problems) _____

      3. Supervisor interview _____

      4. Observation of employee _____

      5. Other local input (e.g., school nurse, co-worker, etc.) _____

      6. Additional information needed: _____

☐ Reasonable Accommodation is feasible and should include:

1. _____

2. _____

3. _____

☐ Reasonable Accommodation is not feasible for the following reasons:

1. _____

2. _____

3. _____

☐ Defer pending additional information.

Disposition:

_____   _____

Director, Health Services   Date
(or school nurse)

Figure 8-7

ADA DECISION TREE

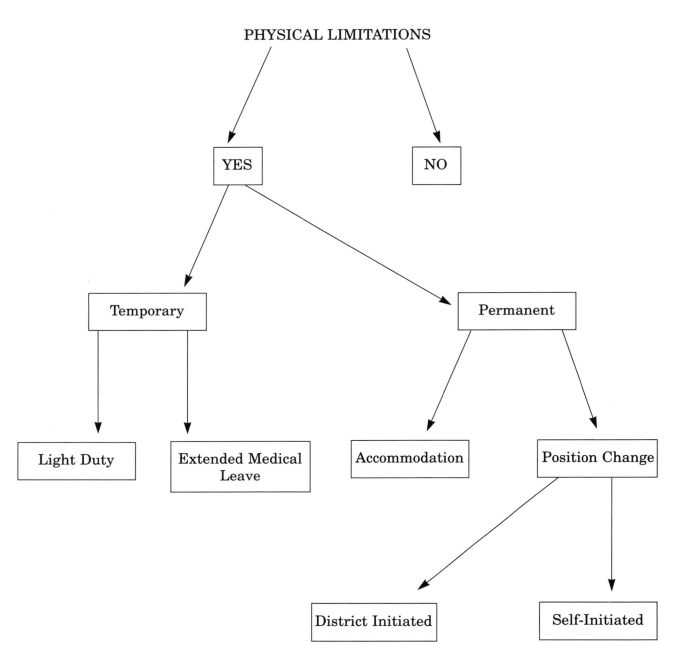

Figure 8-8

EVALUATION OF HIV-INFECTED EMPLOYEE

Date: _____

Case Number: _____ Employee SS Number: _____ DOB: _____

Position: _____

Other Diagnoses: _____

ABILITY TO PARTICIPATE IN INSTRUCTION:

Physical: Is employee too weak or ill to continue?   Yes   No   Unknown

Mental Capacity: Does the employee have memory
impairment or difficulty processing
information?   Yes   No   Unknown

POTENTIAL FOR CONTAGION:

CONFIDENTIALITY: Who should know?   List by Position and Name

1.

2.

3.

4.

RECOMMENDATIONS:

Continue present position   Yes   No

Consider medical leave   Yes   No

Further evaluation needed   Yes   No

(If yes, specify): _____

Accommodations needed:

1.

2.

3.

4.

_____   _____
Signature   Title

Figure 8-9

ACTIVE EMPLOYEE CASE
Health Services

NAME: _____

ADDRESS: _____

SOCIAL SECURITY NUMBER: _____ DATE OF BIRTH: _____

HOME PHONE NUMBER: _____

WORK PHONE NUMBER: _____

EXISTING FILE: YES   NO

REFERRED BY: _____

CURRENT POSITION: _____ BUILDING ASSIGNMENT: _____

REASON FOR REFERRAL: _____

_____

_____

_____

_____

_____

_____

_____

DISPOSITION: _____

_____

_____

_____

_____

_____

_____

_____   _____
      DATE   School Nurse (Or other school health professional)

XC:

Figure 8-10

LETTER TO PHYSICIAN
(Employee Health Problem)

Dear Doctor _____:

Your patient—our employee— _____ has indicated a

health problem. The supervisor feels it is interfering with attendance and/or job

performance.

_____ has signed the enclosed release authorization

for you to communicate with me. It would be helpful, in trying to assist our mutual client, if

you could submit a brief statement on this individual's ability to continue in the current

position; please list any limitations. As well, we would appreciate having your assurance

that this employee does not pose a threat to himself or herself, or to others in the school

setting in terms of physical safety, contagion, or other problem.

Please feel free to submit this in writing, by fax (_____) or by telephone

(_____). I know we both want to do what we can to minimize any

negative impact in the work setting. The information you send will be shared only on a

need-to-know basis.

Sincerely,

Director, School Health Services

(or School Nurse)

Figure 8-11

RESOLUTION
WELLNESS PROGRAM

WHEREAS   the quality of life is directly related to the level of intellectual, emotional, physical, and social well being of the individual; and

WHEREAS   health promotion programs such as those aimed at stress reduction, smoking cessation, weight control, exercise, and the reduction of drug/alcohol use, have the potential to help both school staff and students develop healthy lifestyles; and

WHEREAS   school nurses recognize the importance of a healthy lifestyle for maintenance of an optimum level of wellness throughout life; and

WHEREAS   school nurses have the educational background and skills relevant to wellness programs;

THEREFORE BE IT RESOLVED   that the National Association of School Nurses believes that school nurses should actively support and participate in health promotion programs for both school staff and students; and

BE IT FURTHER RESOLVED   that the National Association of School Nurses believes that school nurses should utilize their professional preparation and skills as health consultants to wellness programs.

National Association of School Nurses
Adopted June 1987

CHAPTER 9

DEALING WITH ADULTS

Chapter 9

DEALING WITH ADULTS
===

You can't go out and teach a community to think
clearly if you can't think clearly yourself.

—Martin H. Fischer (1879–1962)

The effective school nurse must not only master the technical aspects of the profession but also be proficient at people skills. People skills are those behaviors that allow you to accomplish tasks with others—whether they be clients (students, parents), peers (a committee of nurses), or bosses (principals and other administrators). These skills include

- communicating—clearly articulating your goals to others
- listening—understanding the goals of others
- acting—implementing joint projects when common goals exist

Being an effective school nurse depends on convincing others that you and they have common goals, and by working together you can accomplish more than separately. Sounds easy, and it would be if more people understood this pragmatic truth; however, there are enough who don't to make effective cooperation a complex challenge. This chapter will address ways to establish and accomplish common goals with the various groups you work with.

SCHOOL PERSONNEL

School Board Members

School trustees are elected officials who serve without pay. They are answerable to the local citizens, but also are bound by applicable state and federal law. In addition, state departments of education have policies that must be observed. Figure 9-1, "Education Governance," located at the end of this chapter, illustrates a typical state hierarchy of education governance.

Local school board members, in turn, formulate local policies, which may require more, but not less, than state and federal requirements. The superintendent and his or her staff implement these policies.

While you will not often interact directly with school trustees, it is essential that you not incur opposition from them. Knowing the board's priorities for the year and the pet topic of the moment may influence the method or timing for implementing a health-related activity. Of course, certain topics are inherently sensitive: birth control, drug abuse, violence, ethnic tension, and gay teens to name a few. Even though board members may want school staff to deal with these issues, they must be responsive to their constituency.

Principals

Traditionally, school nurses report to the principal. To gain the principal's support, you must demonstrate your contribution to the total education program. Do you reduce absences and out-of-class time? Do you operate in a vacuum as if nothing existed outside the clinic? Focusing health efforts on goals for students (which everyone buys into) will produce the best results.

There is one person who's always right: the boss. The principal is the boss and enjoys almost absolute power. Those who have an autocratic leadership style can be difficult, particularly if they believe they can make health-related decisions personally. Even under these circumstances, a successful school health program can be implemented. Here are some tips.

1. Tie all health activities (even if indirectly) to student attendance and achievement.
2. Use objective data to demonstrate student need.
3. Obtain parent and teacher support.
4. Let the boss take credit for your good idea (or, better yet, make it look like the boss's idea).

It can also be a problem when the principal's leadership style is the opposite—so democratic that all decisions are slow to come or never arrive at all. This sort of non-decision-making boss can stymie almost any project. Part of the inaction may stem from fear of criticism (no decision, no criticism). Strategies for dealing with inaction depend on correct assessment of the reason for it. If it's the fear of criticism, you must demonstrate support for a given activity from the principal's constituents (teachers, students, parents, etc.), and allay those concerns regarding negative opinions. Two other factors that often influence the slow-motion decision maker are

- cost savings (demonstrate that it will be more expensive in the long run *not* to initiate an activity)
- lessening of legal liability (show greater risk is involved if the activity is *not* carried out)

An infinite number of leadership styles exist among principals and these two merely represent the extremes. By keeping one eye on students and the other on politics, you will rarely meet an insurmountable principal. Most, in fact, are supportive.

Teachers

There is absolutely no question that teachers are the most important employees in a school district. What happens for students in the classroom is the heart of education. Class time is sacred except in emergencies. If you lose sight of this truism you are borrowing a very large set of problems. On the other hand, the nurse who respects and protects class time will garner the respect of all teachers. Anything you can do to reduce out-of-class time for major subjects will be appreciated.

Another way you can be perceived as helpful by teachers is to provide classroom management tips—as for the student with attention deficit hyperactivity disorder. Although these activities represent common sense, courtesy, and good nursing practice, they require a conscious and continued effort.

A third facet of teacher relations is dealing with teachers who overrefer to the clinic: Any and all student complaints are sent to you. This is a particular problem during the winter respiratory season. Proactive education of teachers regarding criteria for clinic referrals is a good investment of time. The opposite problem is the teacher who will not let any child leave her or his class. This teacher believes all students are either hypochondriacs or liars. Here again, written guidelines for clinic referrals should be given, with a passing mention of the potential for parent distress should a serious illness be overlooked (e.g., the diabetic student whose headache is due to hypoglycemia).

As with principals, I have taken extreme examples of teacher behavior. Most teachers are cooperative and show good judgment. Don't neglect this group, because they will be your strongest supporters in faculty and PTA meetings.

Special Education Personnel

Teachers of students with disabilities are generally rewarding to work with because their students have more health problems and, thus, a greater need for your expertise. A point of contention sometimes arises when special student procedures are required daily, yet the school nurse is not full time. A few teachers feel it is not their duty to perform tracheal suctioning or administer tube feedings. If a capable teacher aide is assigned to the classroom, this often solves the problem. If not, there are two other options:

- include these duties in the teacher job description and make it clear prior to hiring
- assign the child to another, more willing, teacher

Forcing an experienced teacher to do something she or he resents and has never done before is seldom in a student's best interest.

Special education personnel outside the classroom include a variety of individuals from managers to providers. You will interact with them most often in student review committees where special education candidates are considered. They include educational diagnosticians, psychologists, and occupational therapists. Here the challenge is reaching a consensus about the IEP (individual education plan). As discussed in Chapter 2, the simplest solution for you is to submit a separate IHP (individual health plan).

Personnel at the grass roots level are usually productive to deal with because a specific child is the focus of deliberation. You will sometimes encounter individuals at the administrative level in special education, whose focus is less student-oriented and more legalistic: "The law says . . . policy requires . . ." My response to such a person is: "Laws and policies are created to serve people—in our case, students. The regulation you are quoting doesn't seem to be helping this student. Certainly we don't want to flagrantly break a law, but couldn't we creatively flex it to help the child?"

As in dealing with all adults in the school setting, keep the focus on children! Laws, budgets, and all other considerations are secondary to the needs of the students.

Nurse Peers

You can feel isolated when you are the only health professional on campus. Opportunities for being with other school nurses are often limited to infrequent "administrative" meetings where little networking is feasible. Despite the challenge, interacting with nurse peers is important to professional growth. Some ways to ensure interaction include

- attending national, state, and local conferences
- reading nursing and pediatric journals
- reviewing audio- and videotapes
- urging expanded school district staff development (volunteer to be on a planning committee)
- forming special interest groups (high school nurses for teen parents)
- corresponding with (or calling) colleagues in other cities

The goals of such activities are to grow professionally, to share tricks of the trade, and often, to obtain and provide moral support. In the latter category, sharing frustrations is an important safety valve—essential to maintaining good mental health.

Nurse Aides

Nurse extenders performing the same basic duties come with various labels: nurse aide, nurse assistant, health assistant, clinic helper, health room aide. School nurse groups and school budget personnel have seen the wisdom of freeing nurses from routine tasks to spend more time on professional nursing activities, such as health counseling and health education.

With proper training and supervision, using nurse aides can be a cost-effective option—salaries are usually at the teacher aide level. The challenge is to find good people interested in health and willing to take on more responsibility for a teacher aide salary. A few individuals working elsewhere in schools want to provide health services, but not enough to fill the demand. Three ways of enhancing recruitment are the following:

- Provide salaries above teacher aide level.
- Provide salary increases after a successful first year.
- Build in significant status for the position (through recognition, paid seminar attendance, and other perks).

You must provide adequate performance monitoring, ongoing training, and thorough evaluation for effective use of nurse extenders, especially those who frequently function independently (cover a school when the nurse is not present). Figure 9-2 is an example of a brief yet comprehensive evaluation for a nurse aide.

School principals and other administrators must be made to understand that it is the registered nurse who supervises and determines the appropriate utilization of any unlicensed assistant involved in providing direct health care to students.

Volunteers

The effective use of volunteers requires careful selection and continuous nurturing. Adult clinic volunteers are most often parents of students attending the school. Reasons for using parent volunteers include

- entry point for parent involvement
- public relations (any parent involvement is good for schools)
- educating parents regarding overall school operation
- assisting the nurse with nonprofessional tasks

Parent clinic volunteers should not function in the clinic without supervision (remind the principal that liability reverts to him or her). Take special care to see that volunteers do not have access to confidential data and that sensitive information from students is not repeated, except to the nurse.

Student volunteers are, or should be, used for slightly different reasons. While they can also be helpful nurse extenders, there should be something in it for the student. Whenever possible, select students with an interest in health. It's a golden opportunity to foster this interest and provide career-related information.

PARENTS

Cooperative Parents

The great majority of parents want the best for their children. They may not know how to ask for it but the basic wish is there, particularly when it comes to health care. Even with positive parents, the school must often take the initiative to stimulate involvement. Involved, cooperative parents are the goal and the dream of all school personnel. They must first be invited, then made to feel participatory.

Uninvolved Parents

A significant minority of parents leave everything to the schools—not just education. It is sometimes difficult to know whether this reflects complete trust or merely the path of least resistance. This group is a little harder to get cranked up. You have a unique advantage when you contact uninvolved parents about their child's health; you may be the portal or entry for wider school involvement of such parents.

Difficult Parents

Difficult parents fall into five groups (with some overlap) and include those who

- expect the school to grant every request
- are never satisfied with the status quo
- have hidden agendas that are never discovered
- are looking for financial or other gain through legal action
- don't know what they want, but know it's their "right" as taxpayers to keep the school people jumping

The cause must be identified before corrective action can be taken. When this is not possible, the nurse, principal and other school personnel must be scrupulous in their attempts to do what is, in their professional opinions, best for the child. As the school nurse you will want to communicate more frequently with such parents so they are informed and never surprised by anything that happens with their child. If the parents are litigious, then frequent, objective progress notes of conversations and activities will be necessary.

Dysfunctional Families

Characteristics of the dysfunctional family were discussed in Chapter 5. You will recall the salient features are

- inconsistent messages
- isolated/secretive
- trust violating
- rage/violence
- denial of addictive behavior
- scapegoating
- chaotic

Usually, at least one parent in a dysfunctional family has a diagnosable psychiatric problem (from borderline personality to alcoholism). These are the families from which neglected and abused children come and you must be, first and foremost, the child's advocate.

I recall one eighth grade student with diabetes—we'll call him Mark—who lived with his dysfunctional mother and her boyfriend. Mark required daily insulin shots and was knowledgeable and conscientious about giving them to himself. He had a part-time job after school in order to buy higher protein foods than his mother provided. Mark purchased baloney, cheese, and beans. The mother bought soft drinks, chips, and confections. The mother's boyfriend would eat Mark's food while he was at school. Finally, the school nurse reported this as abuse, and Mark was removed from the home.

Trying to work with dysfunctional families is among the most frustrating and unproductive of the school nurse's activities. You may give up on the family, but you can never give up on the child. Surprisingly often, a child can be salvaged from his or her domestic fate by a few interested school people.

COMMUNITY HEALTH PROFESSIONALS

Physicians

Given the long list of possible joint activities between physicians and schools, it is critical that physician-prescribed care (medications, procedures) be communicated in writing to the school nurse or other official. Telephone orders are acceptable in urgent situations. Do not allow parents to be the sole bearers of physician instructions. They may misunderstand, forget, and over- or understate the doctor's intent. Because of the Nurse Practice Act in most states, school nurses can carry out only physician-prescribed procedures and give only prescription medications.

Here are some guidelines for physicians in communicating with schools (adapted from Nadar, 1993):

- Always inform parents and obtain permission to communicate with the school.
- When contacting a school for the first time, speak to the principal.
- Approach all school personnel as professionals with skills and interests that can complement your expertise and can provide information that you do not have.
- Encourage direct parent-school communication.
- Listen carefully to the concerns and questions of school personnel, and attempt to respond to them.
- Be willing to attend a school meeting, if necessary, to share information or generate management plans.

The advent of faxes has made it easier to communicate with busy physicians.

Agency Personnel

Most school nurses must refer identified problems for treatment. They depend on community health agencies, such as health departments, public clinics, county hospitals, and private agencies in addition to private physicians. Although the usual protocol is to refer to the family doctor, fewer students now have them. Thus, nurse contacts are essential in these community health facilities if students are to receive adequate and timely care. Maintaining good contacts means staying on top of individual names of receiving personnel (it's always best to talk nurse to nurse), referral criteria, waiting time, charges (if any), and other parameters. Most school nurses have developed this skill well, simply because it is so essential to their effectiveness in securing treatment for students.

One issue that warrants special mention is service gaps. For example, there may be inadequate mental health resources, insufficient appointment slots for dental care, or no source of inexpensive glasses for students. Nurses can entice community agencies, corporations, and individuals to work toward ameliorating these problems through financial contributions, volunteerism, and other means. These community development activities are worth a considerable investment of time.

Committees and Advisory Groups

The world seems to need committees. Some are effective; others are a waste of time. If you value your time, you will consider carefully before accepting an invitation to join a committee (if you have a choice). You will also think carefully before forming a committee yourself.

A number of labels are applied to groups of people who function together as committees: task force, advisory council, ad hoc committee, subcommittee, focus group. What they have in common is three or more people trying to make a decision about something. Task forces and ad hoc committees carry out short-term assignments. Standing committees and advisory councils may exist for years. The secret to effective use of people groups is clarity about their function and time lines. One of the reasons short-term committees are effective is that they have a narrowly focused issue to address and a deadline; then they self-destruct. Chronic standing committees tend to lose their focus and develop lives of their own beyond the purpose for which they were created.

I make liberal use of ad hoc committees (if it's a broad issue with community representatives, I give it the loftier title of task force). I use the assignment sheet illustrated in Figure 9-3 to activate the group. The three most important elements are the:

- task description
- end product expected
- ending date

A carelessly conceived task force or committee may end up identifying its creator as the problem.

Committees must meet. Some people love meetings and use them for various purposes other than the assigned task: soapbox for their philosophy, a social event, a vehicle for change (their agenda), and a number of other less than worthy purposes.

The chair of a committee is a tricky role to fill. The chairperson should be chosen for special interest and knowledge in the issue to be addressed, plus an ability to bring people to a consensus. In most cases, the chair should express opinions and vote (if this is necessary). To keep a meeting on task, agendas and time limits are essential. It's also a good idea to have a record of the meeting—not necessarily elaborate minutes. The meeting record can be a few handwritten notes on a form similar to the one shown in Figure 9-4, "Meeting Summary Report."

This simple meeting record serves as a group memory of decisions. There can be no doubt what was decided and what the next steps are. Committees always report to someone, and meeting notes will keep the person receiving the information informed of progress. If the committee is off track, it can be corrected early rather than discovered at the termination of the assignment.

Fringe Practitioners

The number of "health practitioners" has increased dramatically in recent years. Part of the expansion is due to medical specialization. Another part has resulted from lay interest in "holistic medicine" and nonmedicine (self-healing).

The school nurse treads a thorny path in advising parents regarding practitioners not in the mainstream of modern health care: Hispanic curanderos, occupational therapists who provide "sensory integration" exercises for learning disabilities, optometrists who recommend eye exercises for the same condition, chiropractors who have ranged beyond the scope of their licensed practice. The list is long, but you, the school nurse, can be a child advocate and keep the peace with his or her parents if you use this mental checklist:

- Is the treatment of proven effectiveness (beyond a few testimonials)?
- Are there potential side effects?
- How expensive is the treatment?

The most objective evidence available should be presented to the parents. Only when the potential for harm or unnecessary expense is great should you be assertive. For example, it is one thing for an Asian student to receive "coin rubbing" in addition to antibiotics for an ear infection, yet quite another not to receive antibiotics at all.

SPECIAL INTEREST GROUPS

It seems everyone wants to capitalize on the captive audience of school children, whether it be to convey information, do research, or provide a service. For many school districts, this is a tricky area because it is not desirable to alienate important groups. The solution lies in establishing guidelines for evaluating unsolicited requests to perform activities in the school setting. In the health area these requests may range from requests to pass out pamphlets during National Dental Health Week, to requests from podiatrists to screen feet, to clinical research requests from major universities.

One set of criteria for evaluating out-of-district program requests is shown in Figure 9-5, "Approval of Health Programs." Uniform application of pre-established criteria will be accepted by the community as fair.

It is very common for community professionals, such as dentists, to offer to give a class talk on dental health or perform screenings. Unfortunately, they also want to leave their business cards and receive referrals. Such proprietary interests cannot be allowed.

ORGANIZATIONS

The advantages of keeping in touch with national health and education organizations are fairly obvious:

- to keep in touch with current issues relevant to school health
- to obtain support and credibility for local programs by following national standards and recommendations

Only two organizations deal exclusively with health in schools: The National Association of School Nurses and The American School Health Association. The former publishes the *Journal of School Nursing* and the latter the *Journal of School Health*. Both are required reading for school nurses who wish to stay current.

Other organizations that address school health issues are:

- American Nurses Association
- American Academy of Pediatrics
- American Public Health Association
- American Dental Association
- American Psychological Association
- American Psychiatric Association

These organizations are a good source of national data and trends that can be used to support local strategic planning. They also promulgate most of the ethics that health professionals observe—going beyond what state practice laws stipulate.

ADDITIONAL CONCEPTS

Nurses in supervisory roles and those who chair committees or have at least occasional managerial functions need even greater skill in understanding human nature and group dynamics. Two key concepts in this area are

- motivating and structuring willing individuals
- handling difficult people

Motivating

Mounds of research have identified six powerful motivators:

- worthiness of the task
- responsibility
- achievement
- recognition
- growth
- advancement based on accomplishment

These motivators apply to community volunteers and parents as well as full-time employees, although in slightly different ways. Note that financial reward is not on the list. It is not uncommon for individuals to make a financial sacrifice to do something they believe in.

Another essential ingredient is the leader's attitude and enthusiasm, which will be mirrored by group members. Be sure to avoid slipping into negativism—even while dealing with the negative behaviors of others.

Nonteam Players

The basic categories of difficult people include

- the cynic
- the self-proclaimed expert
- the hostile aggressive
- the passive aggressive

A number of excellent management texts provide strategies for dealing with each of these (see Bramson 1981 for an example). The secret to limiting the negative impact of such people is to have a structure that prevents one individual from dominating a group. *Robert's Rules of Order* were promulgated to achieve this at large group meetings. While it's rarely necessary to be so formal, the basic concepts must be observed.

- One person speaks at a time.
- The chair controls the flow of business.
- A vote may be called for by any member.
- More information may be requested by any member.
- Personal attacks are not allowed.

Peer pressure is very effective in suppressing problematic behavior. Creating win-win situations is also important so that the difficult individual doesn't lose face. Despite all efforts, difficult people will sometimes gain the upper hand. When this happens, the individual must be removed or worked around, or the rest of the group must walk away, adjourn, or otherwise end the relationship if anything productive is to be achieved.

The business world has an objective measure of its effectiveness—profit. In the educational setting, the profit is improved student achievement. Maintain focus on this "bottom line."

Management Errors

Brown (1987) mentions thirteen errors that managers make. Eight of these apply in the educational setting:

- Refuse to accept personal accountability.
- Fail to develop and train people.
- Try to control results instead of influencing thinking (manipulate people).
- Manage everyone the same way.
- Concentrate on problems rather than objectives.
- Fail to set standards.

- Condone incompetence.
- Recognize only top performers.

When these errors are converted to their positive corollaries, they become axioms for the manager to live by. The best test for any strategy is: How would I want to be treated?

The most important positive corollary is: Concentrate on objectives (not problems). With written objectives in the hands of all participants, the task-oriented manager can frequently refer to them when the train rolls off the track.

SUMMARY

The brightest, most technically competent school nurse will fall short (often very short) of maximum effectiveness by paying insufficient attention to human relations. Your focus must be on solving people problems. You must be able to bring people of different backgrounds together. You must know when to lead and when to follow—when to listen and when to talk—and, like Kenny Rogers, when to walk.

Not all of these people skills come naturally to most of us, but they can be learned and practiced. None of us should stop learning and growing in this most complex area: understanding one another.

REFERENCES

1. Adams, R. "Physicians and Schools—An Elementary Matter." *Dallas Medical Journal* 80(1):22–24, 1994.

2. Bramson, Robert. *Coping with Difficult People.* New York: Anchor Press/Doubleday, 1981.

3. Brown, Steven. *Thirteen Fatal Errors Managers Make.* New York: Berkley, 1987.

4. Curtin, L. "Designing New Roles: Nursing in the 90s." *Nursing Management* 21(2):7–9, 1990.

5. Douglass, Laura. *The Effective Nurse Leader/Manager.* St. Louis: C. V. Mosby, 1988.

6. Earle, Janice. *How Schools Work and How to Work with Schools.* Alexandria, VA: National Association of State Boards of Education, 1990.

7. Jaco, Paula. The Nurse Executive in the Public Sector. *Journal of Nursing Administration* 24(3):55–62, 1994.

8. Jung, Fred. "Evaluation of a Program to Improve Nursing Assistant Use." *Journal of Nursing Administration* 24(3):42–47, 1994.

9. Kawamoto, Kristi. "Nursing Leadership: To Thrive in a World of Change." *Nursing Administration Quarterly* 18(3):1–3, 1994.

10. Kerfoot, K. "To Manage by Power or Influence." *Nursing Economics* 8(2):117–119, 1990.

11. Mark, Barbara. "Emerging Role of the Nurse Manager." *Journal of Nursing Administration* 24(1):48–55, 1994.

12. *Registered Professional Nurses and Unlicensed Assistive Personnel.* Washington, DC: American Nurses Association, 1994.

13. Sullivan, Eleanor. *Effective Management in Nursing.* Menlo Park, CA: Addison-Wesley, 1992.

14. Umiker, William. *Management Skills for the New Health Care Supervisor.* Rockville, MD: Aspen, 1988.

15. Weaver, S. "First Line Manager Skills." *Nursing Management* 22(10):33–39, 1991.

16. Werner, Emmy. "Overcoming the Odds." *Developmental and Behavioral Pediatrics.* 15(2):131–136, 1994.

17. Wheatley, Margaret. *Leadership and the New Science.* San Francisco: Berrett-Koehler, 1994.

Figure 9-1

EDUCATION GOVERNANCE*

STATE EDUCATION POLICYMAKERS

GOVERNOR **LEGISLATURE**

STATE BOARD OF EDUCATION

STATE DEPARTMENT OF EDUCATION

CHIEF STATE SCHOOL OFFICER

STATE DEPARTMENT STAFF
- Administrative Regulations
- Training
- Technical Assistance
- Monitoring

LOCAL SCHOOL BOARD

LOCAL EDUCATION AGENCY
- Superintendent
- General Staff

SCHOOL BUILDINGS
- Principal
- School Staff

*Adapted from the National Association of State Boards of Education.

Figure 9-2

NURSE AIDE EVALUATION

I. General

	Excellent 4	Good 3	Fair-Poor 2	Unsatisfactory 1
1. Attendance				
2. Appearance				
3. Attitude/adaptability				
4. Safety/housekeeping				
5. Policy observance				
6. Job knowledge				
7. Job performance				
quality				
quantity				
8. Dependability				
9. Initiative/creativity				
10. Personal relations				

II. Specific

	Excellent 4	Good 3	Fair-Poor 2	Unsatisfactory 1
1. Administers basic first aid.				
2. Performs selected screening activities (vision, etc.).				
3. Dispenses prescribed medications.				
4. Records selected student health information; keeps accurate data for monthly reports.				
5. Informs nurse of health counseling and health education needs.				
6. Shares other appropriate health information with nurse and maintains confidentiality.				
7. Performs additional tasks and duties as determined by the nurse.				

Figure 9-3

TASK FORCE/AD HOC COMMITTEE ASSIGNMENT

Name of Committee:

Task / Assignment:

Chair:

Members:

Reports to:

Beginning Date:

Ending Date:

Budget / Clerical Support:

Meeting Site and Frequency:

End Product (written report of recommendations, etc.):

Figure 9-4

MEETING SUMMARY

DEPARTMENT _____

TOPIC _____ DATE _____

Persons Attending:

Absent:

Major Issues Discussed:

_____

_____

_____

_____

Major Concerns:

_____

_____

_____

_____

Decisions/Recommendations:

_____

_____

_____

_____

Next Steps:

_____

_____

_____

_____

Completed by

Figure 9-5

APPROVAL OF HEALTH PROGRAMS
OUT-OF-DISTRICT

The School District is interested in implementing health programs that have the potential for enhancing learning.

Proposed programs should meet at least four of the following seven criteria (starred items are mandatory for all programs):

1. Benefit current or future students (service, education, etc.).

2. Reduce absenteeism.

3. Remove or ameliorate a health barrier to learning.

4. Not increase out-of-class time beyond current health appraisal programs.

5. Provide adequate follow-up of identified health problems.

*6. Meet district and community professional and ethical standards as determined by the Board of Education and the County Medical and Dental Societies or other appropriate professional groups.

*7. No proprietary benefit is derived from the activity.

CHAPTER 10

ENVIRONMENTAL ISSUES

Chapter 10

ENVIRONMENTAL ISSUES

Since life itself is a universally fatal sexually transmitted disease, living it to the full demands a balance between reasonable and unreasonable risk. Because this balance is a matter of judgement, dogmatism has little place. Present preoccupations with health are largely unhealthy as the media constantly draws to our attention hazards to health. Many of these hazards are rare and our individual risk of being harmed is extremely small; in this circumstance they should be ignored.

P. Skrabanek, Follies and Fallacies

School nurses have always had a full plate of responsibilities, yet each year new scientific information comes along to crowd it even further. Environmental health issues are the latest helping in this already abundant feast. As the only health professional in the majority of schools, you play a central role in securing a safe environment. This chapter will cover the essential principles involved in assuming this role. See the NASN "Resolution," Figure 10-1, at the end of this chapter.

HISTORICAL PERSPECTIVE

For centuries humankind has contemplated the ill effects of external forces. In the fourth century B.C., Hippocrates, in his treatise "On Airs, Waters and Places," admonished us to consider the human impact of weather, air, and water quality. The Romans described the devastating effects of lead, often found in high concentration in their pottery. Paracelsus wrote a monograph, published in 1567, devoted to the occupational diseases of miners. The first textbook of occupational medicine, *Diseases of Workers,* was published by Ramazzini in 1713. Yet progress remained slow until after 1900, when "black lung" was again described in miners. Not until the 1960s, however, did medical science begin to understand fully such environmental health hazards as the impact of asbestos on workers in the asbestos industry.

Today a myriad of hazards are being contemplated: air pollution, radiation, sound and mechanical stress, chemical exposures, obscure infectious agents, water and food pollution, allergies and sensitivities, and psychological stress. A new specialty of environmental health has been born. Industrial hygienists and public health officials are breaking new ground in academic institutions, private industry, and government agencies. Experience with asbestos abatement mandates has provided a model for investigation of other potential health hazards. School officials and parents have realized that a safe school environment is not a given, but must be achieved through thoughtful application of scientific information.

MECHANISMS OF INJURY

Technological advances, which have produced "the good life," have concomitantly brought potential hazards to health and safety. Modern society accepts this trade-off. We are surrounded by hazards in our daily life, and some of these risks are accepted matter-of-factly. For example, gasoline is not ordinarily thought of as a hazardous material; few stop to think about its flammable and toxic nature. Fortunately, warnings about smoking and running the car engine when filling the tank reduce the risk to an acceptable level. In other words, most hazardous materials, when handled correctly, can be used safely.

As with any new field, a new terminology develops. Ill effects of environmental hazards on humans are expressed as

- *toxic*—causing damage to living tissue
- *carcinogenic*—promoting malignant tissue growth
- *mutagenic*—chemical or physical agent that disturbs the heredity mechanisms in cells (especially the genes in ova or spermatozoa)
- *teratogenic*—any substance that causes physical or functional defects in the developing embryo
- *irritating*—any chemical that causes a reversible inflammation of living tissue at the site of contact
- *sensitizing*—a chemical that causes a substantial proportion of exposed people to develop an allergic reaction to normal tissue
- *threshold limit value (TLV)*—the safe average permissible exposure limits of airborne substances

Common carcinogens in our environment include formaldehyde, benzene, and asbestos. Carbon tetrachloride and toluene are mutagens, and lead is a teratogen.

The toxic effects of a substance on a particular individual depend on both the chemical and the individual; that is, if an individual is exposed to a series of different chemicals, toxic effects may occur with minute amounts of some substances, but only after large quantities of others. The toxicity of one chemical can be millions or billions of times greater than the toxicity of another. Human variation is not as great. If a particular chemical causes an effect in one individual when a particular amount is administered, it is not likely that an amount a million times less will cause a toxic effect in another individual. While the exact range of human variability is not well established, it is probably closer to a hundredfold than a billionfold.

The concept of *portal of entry* is essential to understanding human toxicity from environmental health hazards. Portals of entry denote the sites at which toxins enter the body. The skin, respiratory tract, and gastrointestinal tract are the primary portals of entry for humans. Many chemicals can be absorbed into the bloodstream from these sites. Once absorbed, a toxin is attacked by the body's metabolic mechanisms. In humans, the liver and the kidneys are the primary detoxifiers, and are consequently often damaged; both are essential to life. The respiratory tract, brain, or unborn fetus may be adversely affected as well.

REGULATORY LEGISLATION AND POLICY

The sixties brought social change, and people changed the way they viewed the world, resulting in an environmental awareness explosion. This increasing awareness of contamination of air, water, and land became a universal concern.

Acid rain, ocean dumping, ozone depletion, and the greenhouse effect forced the U.S. government to realize that environmental pollution went beyond state boundaries and that a national policy supported by legislation was necessary. This led to the passage of seven environmental laws that began a formalized effort toward improving the environment: Clean Water Act, Safe Drinking Water Act, Clean Air Act, Toxic Substances Control Act, Federal Insecticide, Fungicide, and Rodenticide Act, Resource Conservation and Recovery Act, and the Occupational Safety and Health Act.

In 1970, two federal agencies were established: the Environmental Protection Agency (EPA) and the Occupational Safety and Health Administration (OSHA). Their function was to enforce the regulations promulgated under the authority of the seven laws. Although the missions of the two agencies are similar—to reduce chemical exposures that may present a hazard—they cover separate populations. OSHA covers employees in the private sector, protecting their right to a safe and healthful workplace. EPA focuses on the environment and on protecting the public from exposure to toxic substances. The only crossover is the EPA's Worker Protection Rule, which covers public employees performing asbestos abatement, including those in school districts.

As science has advanced, so has the ability to detect chemicals in our environment, in concentrations far less than could have been detected 10 years ago. The relationship between chemical exposures, latency period, and cancer has become clearer. Many chemicals at very low concentrations have been implicated as carcinogens. Earlier concerns centered around exposures in the industrial workplace; then investigators began to look at contaminants in the home and office. A result of this investigation was the discovery that asbestos, radon, and lead were potential problems.

Asbestos

In the late 1970s, EPA's Technical Assistance Program provided school districts with technical information about asbestos and encouraged the districts to identify asbestos within their schools, in the hope that all school districts would voluntarily inspect their buildings; however, not all of them did so. Consequently, on May 27, 1982, the EPA, under the Toxic Substance Control Act, proposed the Asbestos-in-Schools Rule requiring schools to inspect for friable asbestos; collect and analyze samples; notify parents, teachers, and employees of the results; and keep records.

The Asbestos-in-Schools Rule did not require the school districts to take any action. The failure of the rule to address this issue, along with other problem areas, led to the passage by the U.S. Congress of the Asbestos Hazard Emergency Response Act (AHERA). AHERA required schools to inspect their buildings for friable and nonfriable asbestos-containing material. If asbestos was found in such condition as to pose a potential health hazard, the rule called for a response, which might be: repair, removal, enclosure, or encapsulation of the material.

Radon

Like asbestos, radon has been implicated as a cause of lung cancer. Radon is a colorless, odorless gas resulting from the radioactive decay of thorium and uranium, both of which are naturally occurring elements found in low concentrations in rock and soil. Radon has a half-life of 3.8 days, and undergoes further radioactive decay in the lungs, producing isotopes that contribute to the adverse health effects. Radon gas enters buildings through cracks and pores in the foundation. In 1984, extremely high levels found in some homes in eastern Pennsylvania focused national attention on the problem.

In January of 1988, the Indoor Radon Abatement Act was passed by Congress, with the goal of reducing levels of radon inside buildings so that they are no higher than radon levels in the ambient environment. The law authorized the EPA to conduct a study to determine the extent of radon contamination in schools. In late 1988, the EPA recommended that school systems test their buildings for radon. However, at this time there are no regulatory requirements for testing.

Lead in Drinking Water

The health hazards of lead are well documented. They include serious damage to the central nervous system, kidneys, and liver; interference with physical growth; fertility problems; and miscarriages. Children are particularly sensitive to the effects of lead exposure in that their bodies tend to absorb and retain more lead. Studies indicate that low levels of lead intoxication can result in reduced IQ levels, impaired learning and language skills, loss of hearing, reduced attention spans, poor classroom performance, and seizures. Because of the myriad of health problems caused by lead, and the fact that elevated levels of lead have been found in drinking water, the Lead Contamination Control Act (LCCA) was passed in October 1988. The act requires

1. EPA to publish a list of brand and model numbers of drinking water coolers that are not lead free

2. prohibition of the manufacture for sale of water coolers that are not lead free

3. EPA to publish a guidance document and testing protocol to assist schools in detecting lead contamination in their drinking water

4. school districts to identify water coolers that are not lead free, and to repair or remove water coolers with lead-lined tanks

5. notification of school personnel and parents of the results of any testing.

"Sick Building Syndrome"

Escalating energy costs in the 1970s resulted in a focus on energy-efficient buildings that reduced air exchange between the inside and the outdoors, serving to concentrate indoor air pollutants. Although most of the problems have been identified in office buildings, schools often have similar ventilation design, and consequently are capable of producing similar problems, collectively termed *sick building syndrome (SBS)*. Reported symptoms also may be of psychogenic origin or subjectively exaggerated by psychological factors. The prevention or treatment of SBS in modern buildings involves ensuring that the fresh air intake is adequate (more under psychological factors).

The scope of this book does not permit further discussion of specific hazards. See the references and readings at the end of this chapter for more information.

ASSESSING ENVIRONMENTAL CONCERNS

Recognition of environmental hazards requires an understanding of the association between exposure to a toxic substance and the resulting adverse health effect, i.e., the dose-effect relationship.

There are three basic approaches to documenting an environmental health hazard:

1. Measuring toxins in the environment. Air sampling is the most often used technique. The concentration of toxins in the air is compared with standards published by federal agencies and professional organizations, for example, the number of asbestos fibers per cubic meter of air.

2. Epidemiologic approach. This establishes prevalence of a specific health effect on the exposed population and compares it with an unexposed population.

3. Monitoring health effects. This method is especially useful with known toxins causing acute or subacute health effects, for example, pesticides. Such monitoring may include blood tests that detect the toxin or identify adverse effects, such as suppressed red cell enzymes.

Assessment of environmental health hazards is challenging, given current knowledge and the apprehension and subjective overlay that often exist in exposed populations. Adequate evaluation of health effects depends heavily on the availability and accuracy of records: health records and Material Safety Data Sheets (MSDS).* See Figure 10-2. If records are unavailable or unreliable, symptom questionnaires, medical interviews, or diagnostic tests may be needed. Appropriate environmental specialists should be consulted in the design and interpretation of these evaluations.

OVERLOOKED SCHOOL HAZARDS

Many administrators, teachers and students incorrectly assume that the only hazardous chemicals in schools are in science labs. Flammable materials are broadly distributed in art, industrial art, home economics, health, office, custodial and maintenance, athletic, and many other instructional work areas. The same can be said for corrosive chemicals and poisons of various potencies. Chemicals that can produce cancer or birth defects are common in art materials (glazes, paints), office supplies (Liquid Paper, rubber cement), industrial arts, and custodial and maintenance products. Inhalation is the primary route

---

*Manufacturers must develop a MSDS for each hazardous chemical they produce. Employers must have a MSDS for each product containing a hazardous chemical they use.

of exposure to many of these hazardous materials, but some are absorbed through the skin if proper precautions are not followed.

Few employees or students are aware that all photocopy machines produce toxic levels of a "natural gas" if not well ventilated. Even the installation of carpets in classrooms or tarring a roof has produced crises of the first order.

Figure 10-3 lists materials that may be harmful to adults and children by departmental category . Material Safety Data Sheets (MSDS) and labels should always be reviewed and precautions followed prior to the use of any chemical. See Figure 10-4, "Standard Label for Toxic Substance."

PSYCHOLOGICAL FACTORS

When employee or student symptoms suggestive of building-related illness are not readily explained by a toxin, or an irritating or sensitizing substance, you may want to call on your school psychology colleagues or an outside mental health consultant. This section provides a brief overview of the spectrum of building-related "illnesses."

Four major workplace-related psychological disorders can be distinguished (Ryan 1992):

- "sick" or "tight" building syndrome (SBS)
- building-related illness (BRI)
- neurotoxic disorders (NTD)
- mass psychogenic illness (MPI)

These four disorders have several characteristics in common and are not mutually exclusive. Although a number of workers or students may be in the vicinity of an environmental event (unusual odor, chemical, etc.), not all develop symptoms. Individual differences in susceptibility are thought to reflect the presence or absence of specific physiological and psychological characteristics that serve as risk factors.

Sick Building Syndrome

SBS is characterized by five general types of symptoms: mucous membrane irritation (eyes, nose, throat), neuropsychiatric disturbances (fatigue, headaches, dizziness), skin disorders (itching, dry skin), asthma-like symptoms, and unpleasant odor or taste perceptions. Symptoms tend to increase during the day and abate in the evening and on weekends. By definition, these symptoms are not caused by known toxins (e.g., formaldehyde). People in clerical positions who do a great deal of photocopying, who are dissatisfied with their supervisors, and who are generally unhappy at work are at the greatest risk. Smoking, or working in an environment with many smokers, is also associated with more symptoms. SBS, then, is caused by multiple factors and often exaggerated by psychological stressors.

Building Related Illness (BRI)

Unlike SBS, BRI has a known cause with specific symptoms and laboratory findings. The most common diseases are characterized by flu-like symptoms or respiratory distress and include hypersensitivity pneumonitis, humidifier fever, and bacterial pneumonia (e.g., Legionnaire's disease).

Neurotoxic Disorders (NTD)

Exposure to neurotoxic substances like heavy metals (lead, arsenic) and organic solvents (certain paints and cleaning agents) is associated with mood changes, mental and motor slowing, and memory problems. These are rare in the school setting and occur mostly in maintenance departments where neurotoxic chemicals are used on a routine basis. Poisonings are almost always due to improper usage.

In some regions of the country, students inhale organic solvents (e.g., toluene) for the euphoric effect; this originated with glue sniffing, and is a particular problem with Hispanics in the southwestern United States.

Mass Psychogenic Illness (MPI)

Perhaps better called sociogenic illness, this condition is seen in groups of people following a strong (usually harmless) chemical odor or "mystery gas." Symptoms are of a nonspecific physical and psychological nature and cannot be objectively documented (headache, dizziness, fatigue).

Four predictors account for a large number of cases:

• high work intensity/mental strain
• work/home problems
• less than college education
• female gender

Symptoms usually remit following removal from the building. There is usually an "index case" who first develops dramatic symptoms that spread rapidly to others in the same social network. Changing the physical environment (at a very great cost) may have little impact on workers' physical and mental health.

Mental health professionals may use various psychological scales for hysteria, hypochondriasis, and depression to identify individuals at risk for MPI.

SCHOOL NURSE ROLE

The NASN Standards of School Nursing Practice (1993) refer to school nurses as consultants who are actively involved in the establishment and maintenance of a safe and healthy environment within the school district. The increase in federal and state legislation and in the number and types of new environmental health hazard issues has caused the school nurse's role to be expanded.

School Policies

You may be involved in the development of school policies relating to environmental hazards. For instance, because of the documented dangers caused by cigarette smoking, some school districts have instituted a "smoke-free environment" policy. You may help in writing such policies or may be involved in the implementation phase, including the teaching of smoking cessation to students and staff.

Consultant to School Personnel

You are perceived by school personnel and the community as the resident health expert. Questions and concerns regarding recently identified environmental hazards, such as asbestos, radon, and lead in drinking water, may be directed to you. Having information and available resources relating to the short- and long-term effects of these hazards is important. You should know, for example, that asbestos and radon cause no immediately observable health effects. Although lead ingestion may cause lead colic (cramping abdominal pain), it is a very rare symptom; the chronic symptoms of headache, fatigue, or cognitive impairment are more common.

While some school nurses may initially feel uncomfortable in the role of environmental health coordinator, it is essential that you assume this role in school districts where you are the only health professional. Since it is the potential for negative health effects that is being assessed, you are best equipped to synthesize recommendations from outside agencies into a meaningful plan of action with the principal and the school medical advisor.

In larger school districts, the administration will have access to industrial hygienists and other specialists to address environmental concerns. In smaller districts, it may be your responsibility to provide such information. Community resources, such as the Poison Control Center, the Environmental Protection Agency, County Health Department, or the County Extension Office, are among the agencies that you may consult for expert advice. You also need a physician consultant for medical advice relating to environmental issues; this may be the county Health Officer.

Custodial, maintenance, and food service employees are often exposed to hazardous chemicals and products and may be unaware of the potential of these products to cause injury, particularly when inappropriately mixed. Symptoms of exposure to harmful chemicals (coughing, tearing eyes, headaches, dizziness, itching skin, or hand rashes) can be avoided if protective equipment is properly used. It is your responsibility to recommend the provision of safety equipment and to encourage its use.

Chemicals used in such classes as art, science, industrial arts, and cosmetology, and in other technical and vocational classrooms, should be handled and stored properly. The erroneous assumption is often made that chemicals used in these classes are not hazardous. Be aware of the school's chemical safety program, encourage use of appropriate protective equipment, and ensure that emergency procedures are taught. You may also evaluate and monitor chemical disposal procedures and recommend precautions to be used with health hazards. To establish an effective chemical hazard program, some school districts utilize the services of an external consultant. In smaller schools, you may be responsible for this activity or for providing assistance to those who are ultimately responsible.

Office personnel routinely work with products that are flammable, poisonous, carcinogenic, or teratogenic. For instance, fire injuries can occur when duplicating fluids and rubber cement are improperly used or stored. Photocopying and duplicating machines should not be located in the same area, because the vapors from the duplicator solvent may be ignited by electric discharges in the photocopier. Adequate ventilation is important when using photocopying machines. Ozone, a colorless gas, is a strong irritant to the respiratory system, and is produced when oxygen in the air is exposed to the high voltage and ultraviolet light of these machines. Thus, photocopying machines should not be placed in confined closets or in health rooms with limited ventilation, since ozone can produce sore throats, headache, and nausea. Share this information with office personnel and encourage adherence to safety recommendations.

Management of Health Problems

Assessing the symptoms and illnesses that may occur as a result of an environmental exposure, as well as referring the individual to proper medical care, and monitoring the course and treatment of the illness are important functions of a school nurse. A number of indoor air pollutants are generally thought to produce a variety of immediate health effects among building occupants. Biological agents (mold, bacteria, fungus) and chemical agents (formaldehyde, carbon monoxide, ozone, ammonia, tobacco smoke) have been shown to produce headaches, nausea, dizziness, and eye and throat irritation.

Students and staff are often concerned that products such as paint, pesticides, glues, carpets, carpet cleaners, and industrial cleaners may be the cause of a variety of health problems, since they have noticeable odors. An unpleasant odor does not necessarily mean that a health hazard exists. If used and applied properly, such products are not a cause of concern for the healthy individual. There may be some, however, who are sensitive or allergic to a chemical component of these products. Consequently, exposure to such chemicals should be minimized. Figure 10-5 is a suggested letter to parents which can be used prior to painting.

Data Collection, Storage, and Retrieval

Often it is the responsibility of the school nurse to collect data concerning environmental hazards and related health problems. In some school districts school nurses may be responsible for these activities, as well as filing the required reports with monitoring agencies. Written reports and records must be maintained for future reference and protection against legal liability.

A survey of school nurses in a large Texas school district identified the most frequent health-related environmental concern as fumes from indoor painting. Complaints included headaches, nausea, and asthma attacks. On the basis of the survey information obtained, the school administrator in charge of maintenance substituted a paint low in volatile organic compounds. Additionally, when painting was in progress, students and faculty were moved as far away from the paint site as possible and the area being painted was adequately ventilated. An information letter was developed for distribution to staff and parents when buildings were to be painted, explaining that some health problems may be exacerbated by paint fumes. The letter gives the date, time, and exact location of the painting.

To facilitate communication about environmental concerns from the building personnel and parents, send a written report of the concern to the central school administration. The information collected should include the name and address of the location of the complaint, a description of the problem, the length of time that the problem has existed, the observed or reported effect on people, and the number of people affected. See Figure 10-6, "Report of Environmental Concern."

ADMINISTRATIVE CONSIDERATIONS

Perceived budgetary constraints should be weighed against legal liability, Workers' Compensation costs, and public opinion in approaching a potential environmental hazard. An early definitive investigation by a competent environmental specialist is usually the most cost-effective approach. Students, parents, and the news media can be allies in such a proactive approach. Conversely, a sluggish response to a perceived hazard, especially if it includes a defensive posture, may result in an irreparably tarnished public image for the school district and its officials, to say nothing of possibly prolonging a health risk exposure to students and staff.

As in all school matters, the ultimate legal and moral responsibility rests with the board of education and superintendent. At the local level, however, the principal may deal with numerous smaller environmental problems and potential problems, with recommendations from internal and external resources. The most often used resources in the latter category are the local health department and the EPA. Federal agencies concerned with occupational health are listed in Figure 10-7.

SUMMARY

Responsibility for a school environment free of environmental hazards falls primarily to school personnel. To fulfill this responsibility, each must be knowledgeable of potential hazards, federal and state regulatory guidelines, and the role of environmental specialists. You, the school nurse, play a central role in securing a safe environment.

REFERENCES

1. Baselt, R. *Biological Monitoring Methods for Industrial Chemicals.* Littleton, MA: PSG Publishing Co., 1988.

2. Bearg, D. *Indoor Air Quality and HVAC Systems.* Boca Raton, FL: Lewis Publishers, 1992.

3. Blumenthal, D. *Introduction to Environmental Health.* New York: Springer Publishing, 1985.

4. Centers for Disease Control. "Guidelines for Investigating Clusters of Health Events." *Morbidity and Mortality Weekly Report* 39 (No. RR-11):1–21, 1990.

5. Environmental Protection Agency. *A Guide to Indoor Air Quality.* Washington, DC, 1988.

6. Freeman, S. *Injury and Litigation Prevention.* New York: Van Nostrand Reinhold, 1991.

7. Friedman, G. *Primer of Epidemiology.* New York: McGraw-Hill, 1980.

8. Hansen, D. (ed.). *The Work Environment.* Chelsea, MI: Lewis Publishers, 1991.

9. Hernberg, S. *Introduction to Occupational Epidemiology.* Boca Raton, FL: Lewis Publishers, 1992.

10. Igoe, J. "Environmental Health: The Physical Environment." In *Principles and Practice of Student Health* Vol. 2, pp. 369–375. Oakland, CA: Third Party Publishing Co., 1992.

11. Kamrin, M. *Toxicology.* Chelsea, MI: Lewis Publishers, 1988.

12. Legator, M. *The Health Detective's Handbook: A Guide to Investigation of Environmental Health Hazards by Nonprofessionals.* Baltimore: Johns Hopkins University Press, 1985.

13. Levy, B. *Occupational Health: Recognizing and Preventing Work-Related Disease.* Boston: Little, Brown, 1988.

14. McCunney, R. (ed.). *Handbook of Occupational Medicine.* Boston: Little, Brown, 1988.

15. Murdock, B. *Environmental Issues in Primary Care.* St. Paul: Minnesota Department of Health, 1991.

16. Pope, A. (ed.). *Indoor Allergens: Assessing and Controlling Adverse Health Effects.* Washington, DC: National Academy Press, 1993.

17. Rea, W. *Chemical Sensitivity.* Boca Raton, FL: Lewis Publishers, 1993.

18. Roeser, R. "Implementing an Industrial Hearing Conservation Program in the Schools." *Journal of School Health* 53(7):69–72, 1983.

19. Ross, C. *Computer Systems for Occupational Safety and Health Management.* New York: Marcel Dekker, 1991.

20. Ryan, C. "Dysfunctional Buildings or Dysfunctional People: An Examination of the Sick Building Syndrome and Allied Disorders." *Journal of Consulting Clinical Psychology* 60(2):220–224, 1992.

21. Thompson, G. *Concise Manual of Chemical and Environmental Safety in Schools,* Vol. 1. Philadelphia: J. B. Lippincott, 1989.

22. Thompson, G. *Written Hazard Communication Program for Schools and Colleges.* Philadelphia: J. B. Lippincott, 1989.

23. Tucker, W. "Sources of Indoor Air Contamination." New York: *Annals of the New York Academy of Sciences,* Vol. 641, 1992.

24. U. S. Consumer Product Safety Commission. *School Science Laboratories: A Guide to Some Hazardous Substances.* Washington, DC, 1984.

Figure 10-1

RESOLUTION FOR A HEALTHFUL
SCHOOL ENVIRONMENT

WHEREAS: a healthful school environment is an essential part of the learning process for both the student and staff not only as a requirement for safety, but also to develop student attitudes which value a healthy lifestyle, and

WHEREAS: a healthy school environment includes an atmosphere free from pollution such as: tobacco smoke, asbestos; radon; fumes from paint; and the exhaust from mechanical equipment; and

WHEREAS: a healthy school environment is one free from sanitation problems such as faulty plumbing, lead or other chemicals in the water, nonhygienic drinking and bathroom facilities; and

WHEREAS: a healthy school environment is safe for learning, working, and playing, free from defective or poorly maintained equipment, hazardous wiring, dangerous playgrounds, improperly maintained laboratory and vocational equipment and facilities, inadequate lighting, and unacceptable noise levels; and

WHEREAS: school nurses have knowledge and skills in the areas of public health and safety, disaster planning, sanitation, and hygiene;

THEREFORE, BE IT RESOLVED that the National Association of School Nurses recommends that school systems establish and maintain a healthful school environment; and

BE IT FURTHER RESOLVED that the school nurse, as an advocate for students, staff, and community should continue to monitor the school environment and actively advocate for student and staff safety.

National Association of School Nurses

Adopted June 1991

Figure 10-2

CATEGORIES OF A TYPICAL MATERIAL SAFETY DATA SHEET—MSDS

Common Name

Physical/Chemical Characteristics

Emergency First Aid

Hazardous Ingredients

Fire and Explosion Hazards

Health Hazard Data
> overexposure effects
> inhalation
> eyes
> skin
> TVL in air

Reactivity Data

Spill, Leak, and Waste Disposal

Personal Protection

Storage and Containers

Precautionary Label

Environmental Risks

Emergency Phone Number(s)

Figure 10-3

SCHOOL MATERIALS THAT MAY BE HARMFUL

ART MATERIALS
- paints and solvents
- drawing inks
- dyes
- pottery clay (silica)
- resins, dusts
- printing solvents and inks
- wood preservatives
- aerosol sprays
- glues and adhesives
- permanent markers

INDUSTRIAL ARTS
The diversity of hazards in woodworking, autobody repair, photography, cosmetology and electronics shops in schools is too broad and too specialized for a detailed list. The classes, however, are similar and include
- flammables
- corrosives
- poisons
- carcinogens
- mutagens
- teratogens

OFFICE AREAS
- asbestos
- fiberglass
- formaldehyde
- photocopy toner
- ozone
- radon
- tobacco smoke
- duplicator solvents

CUSTODIAL AND MAINTENANCE
- floor finisher (xylene)
- mineral spirits
- paint remover (benzene)
- shellac/varnish
- spray paint (acetone, toluene)
- turpentine
- ammonia
- bleach
- Drano (sodium hydroxide)*
- toilet bowl cleaner
- cleansing powder

* Mixing of acid (bleach) and basic (Drano) cleaning substances results in strong heat and toxic fume-producing reactions.

Figure 10-4

STANDARD LABEL FOR TOXIC SUBSTANCE

ACETONE

DANGER

FLAMMABLE LIQUID

TOXIC IF INHALED OR INGESTED

AVOID PROLONGED CONTACT WITH SKIN

HARMFUL TO EYES

TOXIC TO NERVOUS SYSTEM

Work in well-ventilated area.

Avoid fire and other sources of ignition.

Avoid prolonged contact with skin.

Acme Solvents, Inc.
123 Main Street
Dallas, Texas 75225

Figure 10-5

SUGGESTED LETTER TO PARENTS PRIOR TO PAINTING IN SCHOOLS

Dear Parent:

In the near future, your school will be receiving a much needed coat of paint. The paint used is a low odor enamel. Studies by the Environmental Protection Agency have confirmed the safety of this product.

Certain paints may aggravate asthma or allergies. If your child has such a sensitivity, please submit a physician's statement to me or the school nurse.

If there are other health circumstances that need addressing, contact me for advance consideration.

Yours truly,

Principal

SUGGESTED LETTER TO PARENTS PRIOR TO PAINTING IN SCHOOLS

Estimados Padres:

En un futuro cercano, su escuela va a ser pintada nuevamente. La pintura que se va a usar es un "enamel" de olor mínimo. Estudios hechos por la Agencia para la Protección del Medio Ambiente ha confirmado la seguridad de este producto.

Algunas pinturas pueden empeorar el asma ó las alergias en algunas personas. Si su hijo/hija es una de estas personas, hága el favor de darme ó a la enfermera de la escuela un certificado médico.

Si hay algunas otras circumstancias médicas sobre las cuales nosotros debemos saber, póngase en contacto conmigo para dar adelantadamente consideración a su pedido.

Sinceramente,

Director

Figure 10-6

REPORT OF ENVIRONMENTAL CONCERN

Where: _____
                 Name and Address of Location

Problem statement:

Length of time that this has been a problem:

Number of people affected:

Observed or reported effect on people:

Investigative or corrective measures employed:

Suggestions for alleviating the problem:

Reported by _____ Telephone _____

Date _____

Figure 10-7

FEDERAL AGENCIES CONCERNED WITH OCCUPATIONAL HEALTH

1. Environmental Protection Agency (EPA)
    Consult "Government" pages of local telephone directory for nearest regional office, e.g.
        Region I
        John F. Kennedy Federal Buillding, Rm 2203
        Boston, MA 02203
        Telephone: (617) 565-3715

2. National Institute for Occupational Safety and Health (NIOSH)
        4676 Columbia Parkway
        Cincinnati, OH 46226
        Telephone: (513) 841-4382 or (800) 356-4674

3. Occupational Safety and Health Administration (OSHA)
        U. S. Department of Labor
        200 Constitution Avenue, N.W.
        Washington, D.C. 20210

    Consult "Government" pages of local telephone directory for nearest regional office, e.g.:
        Region II
        1515 Broadway (1 Astor Plaza), Room 3445
        New York, NY 10036
        Telephone: (212) 944-3432

4. National Pesticide Hotline (800) 535-PEST

5. Child and Maternal Health Clearinghouse
        (Publications on lead poisoning) (202) 625-8410

6. National Institutes of Health
        Cancer Hotline (800) 422-6237

CHAPTER 11

CLINICAL RESEARCH AND PILOT PROGRAMS

Scientific Method

The Steps in Clinical Research

Pilot Projects

Ethical Considerations

Funding Research and Pilots

Publishing Research Findings

Research Survival Tips

Summary

Glossary

References

Chapter 11 Figures:

Chapter 11

CLINCAL RESEARCH AND PILOT PROGRAMS

A collection of facts is no more science than a
heap of stones is a house.

—*Lewis Thomas*

Clinical research is the systematic study of people as they interact with their environment. It allows us to advance knowledge by looking carefully at cause and effect in given situations. Sharing the fruits of our investigations keeps us from reinventing the wheel in our local setting. Reviewing the various scientific literatures (nursing, medicine, psychology, education, etc.) allows us to learn from the successes and failures of others.

This chapter will deal with a few basic concepts of the scientific method applied to experimental and descriptive clinical research. It should allow you, the school nurse, to understand published research better and to design studies that will answer questions relevant to your unique practice setting. As Vaughan (1994) has said, "Without the ability to communicate discoveries to our fellow human beings, we would be condemned to endless rediscovery."

The generally accepted priorities for nursing research are listed in Figure 11-1, located at the end of this chapter. Review them now.

SCIENTIFIC METHOD

The heart of the scientific method is the reproducible experiment: evaluating the effect of A on B. The B variable is called the outcome variable (or dependent variable). It is observed to see how it changes as a result of A. The A variable, or independent variable, can be controlled or manipulated to see if its presence effects a change in B. Does a cause and effect relationship exist? Figure 11-2 lists the types of variables and their synonyms. For instance, if A is an antihypertensive medication, we want to know if it lowers blood pressure (B).

In good clinical studies there are many subjects (the patients being studied). When the effect (dependent variable) we are seeking to measure is small or subtle, the study may require hundreds of subjects and sophisticated statistical methods to detect significant changes. The conclusion of the medication study above might read: The drug Loflow lowered the mean diastolic pressure of the study group by 12 mmHg [± 4 mmHg] as compared with the control group.

Types of Research

There are a number of ways to slice the research pie when classifying types. If you want only two pieces, you call them quantitative and qualitative. If you want four pieces, you call them experimental, quasi-experimental, descriptive, and exploratory.

At this point, you may want to start referring to the glossary at the end of the chapter should you come across an unfamiliar term. But, let's deal with a few basic terms in the text. We'll start by defining the types of research we've just mentioned.

- *descriptive:* Observes, describes and classifies phenomena in the nursing profession (e.g., health beliefs, time patterns of temperature readings).

- *exploratory:* Takes descriptive research a step further by establishing the dimensions of a phenomenon, the manner in which it is manifested and other factors with which it is related (e.g., what influences are linked to a person's health beliefs?).

- *experimental:* The most rigorously organized type of clinical research in which the dependent variable can be measured and other variables controlled or their effect accounted for. Such studies usually have large numbers of subjects and the data collected are evaluated by sophisticated statistical methods. This research requires a random selection of study subjects and a control group.

- *quasi-experimental:* A study in which the subjects are not randomly assigned but the researcher can manipulate the independent variable and exercise certain controls.

Figure 11-3 illustrates the degree of investigator control in each of the four types of research. In descriptive and exploratory studies, the researcher makes no changes in the variables, and thus, has little or no control.

The term *nonexperimental research* refers to studies in which the researcher collects data without introducing any changes. (See glossary for retrospective studies and ex post facto design.)

Limitations of Research

The scientific approach is an extremely powerful tool for helping us to understand the world we live in and to solve many practical problems. But our respect for the powers of the scientific approach needs to be tempered by knowledge of its fallibility: the findings from research studies are not always right. That is why it is important for consumers of research to understand the trade-offs and decisions that investigators make and to evaluate the adequacy of those decisions.

Virtually every research study contains some flaw. Perfectly designed and executed studies are unattainable. In most situations, the best methods are expensive and time consuming. Even when tremendous resources are expended, there are shortcomings. This does not mean that small, simple studies are of no value. It means that no single study can ever definitively prove or disprove a researcher's hunches. Each completed study adds to a body of accumulated knowledge. If the same question is posed by several researchers, each of whom obtains the same or similar results, increased confidence can be placed in the answer to the question. This is termed *reproducibility*.

Alternative Inquiry

One of the major obstacles we confront in conducting studies using the scientific model is the complexity of the subjects: humans. Each human is unique in personality, social environment, mental capacities, values, lifestyle, and health status. It is difficult for the scientific approach—which typically focuses on only a small part of the human experience—to capture this complexity. This limitation has led some nurse researchers to reject the traditional model of scientific research.

An alternative model of inquiry has emerged that has its intellectual roots in the philosophic tradition known as *phenomenology*. The phenomenologic approach rests on different assumptions about the nature of humans and how that nature is understood. Phenomenologists emphasize the inherent complexity of humans and their ability to shape and create their own experiences. Investigators in the phenomenologic tradition place an emphasis on understanding the human experience as it is lived, through the collection and analysis of narrative, subjective materials. Phenomenologists believe that a major limitation of the traditional scientific approach is that it is reductionist, that is, it reduces human experience to a few concepts under investigation, and those concepts are defined by the researcher rather than emerging from the experiences of the study subjects.

Both the phenomenologic and the more traditional scientific approaches represent valid and important models for the study of nursing problems. I have devoted more attention to methods normally associated with the traditional scientific approach because most nursing studies employ this method.

THE STEPS IN CLINICAL RESEARCH

Figure 11-4 summarizes the sequence of steps in research.

Finding a Worthy Topic

A review of several texts on nursing research reveals that current topics of interest fall into six general categories:

- compliance with prescribed treatment
- promotion of positive health behaviors
- groups at risk of specific health problems
- nursing process or clinical judgments
- minority groups
- holistic nursing situations

The last category is attractive to nurses who believe that the phenomenological approach is often more revealing than the scientific approach. Studies in this area have focused on phenomena such as parenting, health-seeking behaviors, lifestyle management in the chronically ill, and ethical decision-making behaviors of nurses.

Knowing that these are the areas of study being published in current nursing journals may give you some ideas. Look for a research project with a meaningful clinical question, the answer to which will be useful to you and others—not merely of academic interest: what's referred to as "so what?" research.

Knowing What's Been Done

You must know what's been published in your area of research interest before you finalize the research questions and design the details. Why? Because your question may already have been answered. Even if it hasn't, you'll gain valuable insight by learning the approaches others have taken in pursuing a similar problem.

Finding out what's been done involves reviewing the literature. Each branch of health care has its own published literature and sometimes its own computer data base: Medline, Psychological Abstracts, and ERIC (Education Resources Information Center). Two specific to nursing are

- Cumulative Index of Nursing and Allied Health Literature (CINAL)
- International Nursing Index

Both are published monthly in hard copy and are available annually on compact disks (CD-ROM).

The easiest way to do a literature search is to go to the nearest health sciences center or school of nursing and ask for assistance in doing a computer search of the published literature on your topic. You must have two key words to cross reference and may want to add a third or fourth qualifier to shorten the search. Achieving a narrow focus is essential to a useful literature search. For instance, if your study sought to determine compliance of asthmatic students with their medical regimens you would not want to review the entire literature on asthma; there would simply be too much. If you cross-referenced "asthma" with "school age children" and "treatment," the focus would be narrowed considerably. A fourth qualifier of "compliance with medications" might narrow it too much, but you could begin there to see how many references were generated.

If you are located near a large health sciences center library, there are some attractive options available:

- phone-in requests
- faxing of results
- billing for the service

With the above features, I am usually able to get the information I need within two working days. This is a far cry from taking your index cards to the library and sitting down with the *Index Medicus* for hours.

Ask for the 50 most recent references plus abstracts (English language only). After reviewing the abstracts, you will have a good idea which articles you need to read in their entirety. This means another trip to the library unless you are willing to pay for "pull and copy" service by which articles can be mailed to you. Also, don't forget that each article is a good source of additional references that may not have surfaced in your computer search (different data bases review different journals).

Finally, the newest entries in the computer data base are two to three months old due to entry lag time, so you will probably want to review the last few issues of certain journals on the library shelves.

Having accomplished all this, you should be able to answer these questions about your research topic:

1. Has this been done before?
2. Would it be of interest to colleagues and journal readers?
3. Do I know enough to design a doable research project that will answer an important clinical question?

Designing a Study

Let's say you have been approached by an area hospital or university that wants to study the effect of inhaled steroids on absences in elementary students with asthma. They tell you they would like to have at least 50 study subjects and 50 controls (with 35 and 30, respectively, being the minimum acceptable). You identify all schools in your district with 10 or more students who have moderate to severe asthma and develop a list:

School	Students with Asthma
A	30
B	12
C	23
D	12
E	10
F	35
G	22
H	15
I	10
J	40
K	32

In addition to the hospital's request, you want to limit the study to as few schools as possible. Since the schools are ethnically and socioeconomically balanced, you select the four schools with the largest number of students with asthma and assign them thus:

Study Group	Controls
School J = 40	School A = 30
School K = 32	School F = 35
72	65

A consulting researcher tells you that it would be better to have half the students in each school serve as controls and study the other half, ensuring that both groups are in essentially the same environment. Within each of the four schools you designate study subjects as odd numbered (from an alphabetical list of the students with asthma) and controls as even numbered.

Selecting study subjects is one of the most important aspects of designing a research project; this is known as *sampling*. See Figure 11-5. The term *random assignment* means that each member of a population group has an equal chance of being assigned to the study group. In our asthma study, the even-odd sorting approximates randomization. Without random assignment, selection bias is said to be present (see glossary).

The next step is designing the protocol that will describe the management of study and control subjects. This is not difficult, but it must be detailed and ensure that both groups are treated as nearly alike as possible, especially if subjects and controls are able to observe and talk to each other in the course of other school activities. This is accomplished by a *blind study* which ensures that subjects don't know what group they are in. In blind studies where a medication is administered, it is desirable to use a placebo with the control group to avoid a

Hawthorne effect (see glossary) in the treatment group. Figure 11-6 is a summary form for a research protocol.

Collecting Data

In our study, data collection means securing the numbers called for in the protocol. Without going into detail, it would include such items as student absences, illnesses, number of treatments with inhaled steroid medication, peak flow meter readings, hospitalizations, and medication compliance on weekends.

The simplest type of research involves documenting the values or beliefs of a target population. Questionnaires and interviews are the traditional instruments for collecting such data. Figure 11-7 lists the data collection approaches that can be used in self-report studies. Figure 11-8 contrasts the advantages of questionnaires vs. interviews. The latter, of course, are more time consuming but have greater potential for unexpected findings.

Analyzing Data

This is the part that most of us need help with—time to call your friendly statistician. It is neither feasible nor necessary to memorize statistical formulas, but it is essential to understand the concepts of *probability value* and *statistical significance*. (see glossary). Both relate to chance occurrences. The bottom line of any research is to determine the likelihood that your results occurred by chance. To delve deeper into this important topic, read Denise Polit's book, *Essentials of Nursing Research* (see Chapter 11 references).

Several computer software packages are available to perform a number of calculations on entered data to determine statistical significance.

Drawing Conclusions

Again, you will need to rely on your statistical consultant to tell you when the data show that the study group was significantly different (more than would be expected by chance) from the control group. Figure 11-9 outlines some types of errors in research.

Even in experimental studies, conclusions and inferences can be drawn "beyond the numbers"—conclusions that only you, as the involved health professional, can reach. A variable not addressed in the protocol may surface. For instance, you may discover that several of your Hispanic parents have taken their children with asthma to a curandero and received herbs as treatment. Beyond the possible effect on study results, it is important information for managing Hispanic asthmatics in the future.

PILOT PROJECTS

When you are contemplating a change in the delivery of health services, such as a new procedure, it is always better to confirm the benefits and discover the problems on a small scale first. This will smooth out the rough spots and prevent large-scale (schoolwide, or districtwide) snafus, or it may convince you that the idea should not be implemented. For instance, you may be considering placing peak flow meters in all schools for use by the school nurses in order to better monitor students with asthma. You want to know if this is feasible and cost-effective. You select three or four nurses to pilot its use for a semester. Looking at the following issues will give you some relevant clinical information:

- Can accurate use of the peak flow meter be mastered by all nursing staff?
- Are peak flow meter readings helpful in establishing more specific referral criteria?
- Are many students with asthma already using the instrument at home?
- Do physicians and parents support the instrument's use?
- Does it reduce nurse time in evaluating a student who may be in trouble?
- Does it reduce inappropriate referrals?
- What age student can use the peak flow meter with consistent accuracy? (Falsely low readings are more common in the very young due to lack of maximum effort.)

These and other questions can be easily answered in a pilot. If all looks promising at the end of the pilot, the information gained will also help formulate protocols for wider implementation.

Simpler pilots can be used to field-test new forms or perhaps to see if the portability of laptop computers might be useful to nurses who have two or more schools.

What appears to be a good idea in theory may prove to be of little value in practice. Seldom are we able to predict all the problems that might be encountered in implementing a new idea. A pilot is the answer. Again, small-scale failures prevent large-scale embarrassment and will enhance your reputation as a thoughtful innovator rather than one who impulsively latches on to each new fad or piece of technology.

Sometimes pilots merely let you know that full scale quasi-experimental research is needed to answer the relevant questions. Pilots rarely fail to give you essential information.

ETHICAL CONSIDERATIONS

Clinical research requires the rigorous protection of the rights of the study subjects. Informed consent, confidentiality, and anonymity are at the core of ethical research. They are concepts well known to school nurses but the documentation to establish their presence is ever changing and becoming stricter. All universities and teaching hospitals have human rights committees or institutional review committees that routinely review research proposals. Some school districts have them as well.

Another entitlement of study subjects is the right to freedom from harm. In the inhaled steroid research described above, you might encounter an ethical dilemma if most of the study group experience improvement in their asthma, while many in the control group are getting worse. Are you withholding an important treatment from controls? This is a clinical judgment that should be made with the managing physician of each control subject. If a physician thinks the patient (in the control group) could benefit from inhaled steroids, you would be obligated to drop that student from the study. If several physicians agree concerning their patients, you might be obligated to abort the study. In either event, valuable information has been gained.

FUNDING RESEARCH AND PILOTS

Pilots are traditionally executed with existing in-house resources—"on a shoestring." Full-scale research usually requires special funding and can get expensive. Schools of nursing or teaching hospitals are often interested in cooperative research and may share funding. In some cases, private philanthropy can be a funding source.

Also, medical equipment houses and pharmaceutical companies may be willing to bankroll your project. In the asthma study described, a drug company might be willing to provide its inhaled steroid product free of charge along with the peak flow meters. If you're really serious about research, you may wish to write a formal grant for federal or state funds.

PUBLISHING RESEARCH FINDINGS

If you complete a research project and the findings are significant (a difference between study and control groups), you may have a publishable article that your peers would benefit from reading. Your statistical consultant, perhaps at a school of nursing, can help you determine the level of statistical significance or probability value (e.g., $p < .05$).

The next step is to pick the journal you wish to target. The *Journal of School Nursing (JSN)* and the *Journal of School Health (JOSH)* are two good prospects. Read their "guidelines for authors" in a recent issue. These guidelines will address the types of articles sought, and the procedures for submitting, including format and style, manuscript length, and other specifications. See Figure 11-10. If your study does not represent full-blown research, it may qualify for the section, "Health Service Applications," in JOSH or another journal.

Graphics (charts and tables) are essential to publishing good research. Show your results clearly in tabular form to make them comprehensible at a glance. The narrative text should amplify these data.

The conclusion section is the most important. Far too many authors draw conclusions that are not supported by their data. Keep it objective. If you want to project or generalize, clearly identify what you are doing—and, by all means, acknowledge the limitations of your study.

Most scientific journals are peer reviewed, or refereed; that is, two or more reviewers provide feedback to the editor regarding the publishability of your article. Editor responses may include

- rejection of the article
- acceptance with designated changes
- instructions to revise and resubmit

Most journals do not accept simultaneous submissions.

Here are a few tips in writing your article:

- Write the conclusion first (if you don't have a relevant one, the rest won't matter).
- Write the introduction next to establish why the study was important. You want to convince the potential reader that the results will be useful. (Otherwise your reader may not read past the introduction.)
- Third, write the abstract. This is a summary of the introduction and conclusions—usually about 50 to 150 words.

Now that you know where you're headed, make an outline of the body of the report and proceed to write the text, leading logically toward the conclusion.

Remember that negative results are rarely published. If you show no difference between study subjects and controls, no one will care. (This does not apply to descriptive or exploratory research in which you are merely establishing conditions or belief of your subjects.)

RESEARCH SURVIVAL TIPS

Planning

1. Search the literature. Most scientists consider it a serious handicap to investigate a problem in ignorance of what is already known.
2. Abstract published research. Useful experience can be gained by writing abstracts of published articles. You will become familiar with the worst faults that arise in reporting scientific work and learn to write concisely.
3. Avoid either undue neglect of or undue respect for statistics; know when to consult a statistician.

4. Attend scientific conferences; it is a valuable experience for budding researchers. The annual research sessions of the American School Health Association offer one example.

5. Attend occasional special lectures given by eminent scientists. They can be a rich source of inspiration.

6. Know your own biases.

7. Break the research problem down into several formulated questions; look for gaps in the present knowledge, and differences between reports.

8. Formulate a hypothesis to explain the phenomena under investigation. From the hypothesis certain consequences can usually be proved or disproved by the collection of further observational data.

9. Make a schedule or Gantt chart of sequential activities that must occur. See Figure 11-11.

Execution

1. Have the experimental and control groups as similar as possible in all respects except that of the one factor under investigation.

2. Consider a pilot experiment to obtain tentative results before a large-scale experiment (when time or money are prohibitive).

3. Make sure your research is reproducible (can be repeated by other investigators).

4. Do your best to control all variables except the independent variable.

Assessment

1. Complete intellectual honesty is the first essential in research.

2. When there is a possibility that subjective influences will affect the assessment of results, it is important to obtain objectivity by making sure that the person judging the results does not know to which group each individual belongs (a "blind" observer).

3. Take statistical analysis into account when the experiment is being planned, or the results may not be worth treating statistically.

4. Acknowledge the impossibility of obtaining exactly similar groups.

5. Overestimate the number of subjects required to ensure that "dropouts" don't put you below the number needed for a decisive result.

6. Use common sense in interpreting results after the statistical analysis is completed.

7. Use caution in drawing conclusions as to how generalizable the results are.

8. Never publish investigations that merely fail to substantiate the hypothesis. (Inability to demonstrate a supposition experimentally does not prove it is incorrect.)

Chance

1. Watch out for the unexpected; numerous discoveries in the health field have been accidental (serendipitous).
2. Do not be so obsessed with your hypothesis that you miss or neglect anything not directly bearing on it.

SUMMARY

Studies with true experimental design are difficult to carry out in the school setting without adequate funding and access to statistical expertise. Nevertheless, quasi-experimental and descriptive studies are doable and can significantly advance the knowledge base of school health. Descriptive studies that survey students, parents, and school personnel yield valuable information about the effectiveness of intervention strategies as well as reveal the beliefs and feelings of these individuals.

Research need not be an abstract academic exercise. It often corrects erroneous assumptions we make about our consumers and causes our future efforts to be more productive. The use of schools as research sites is on the rise. Even if you never do research yourself, you should be able to critically evaluate the research published in nursing journals.

GLOSSARY

Applied research	Research conducted to generate knowledge that can be used in practical settings without undue delay.
Attrition	Loss of subjects during a research study.
Basic research	Research designed to formulate theory rather than to be utilized for immediate application.
Blind study	The data collectors know whether subjects are in the experimental or control group, but the subjects do not know. See *double blind study*.
Chi-square	A statistical method used with data to test group differences. Symbol = X^2.
Cohort study	Research examining specific intact subpopulations as they change over time.
Confounding variables	Those phenomena that have an effect on the study variables but are not the object of the study.
Control group	The group in experimental research that does not receive the experimental condition or treatment.
Convenience sampling	Involves the enrollment of available subjects as they enter the study until the desired sample size is reached.
Correlation	The strength of the quantifiable relationship between two or more variables.
Crossover	The reversal of experimental conditions; the treatment or study group and the control group are switched.
Dependent variable	The outcome variable that is observed for change as the independent variable is manipulated by the researcher.
Descriptive research	Research that yields descriptive knowledge of population characteristics and relationships among them.
Double blind study	Experimental strategy in which neither the subjects nor those who collect the data know which subjects are in the experimental group and which subjects are in the control group.
Ethnography	A naturalistic research design concerned with the description and interpretation of cultural patterns of groups and understanding of the cultural meanings people use to organize and interpret their experiences.
Experimental design	The classic two-group design in which subjects are randomly selected and randomly assigned to

either an experimental or a control group condition. Before the experimental condition, all subjects are pretested or observed on a dependent (outcome) measure. In the experimental group, the independent variable or experimental condition is imposed, and it is withheld in the control group. Subjects are then posttested or observed on the dependent variable after the experimental condition.

Experimental group	The group in experimental design that receives the experimental condition; the study subjects.
Explanatory research	Research designed to predict outcomes.
Exploratory research	Studies conducted in natural settings with the purpose of discovering phenomena, variables, theory, or combination thereof.
Ex post facto design	Nonexperimental design in which the phenomena of interest have already occurred and cannot be manipulated in any way; same as retrospective study.
Extraneous variable	Uncontrolled variable outside the purpose of the study that influences the study's results; same as confounding variable.
Face validity	A subjective method for determining validity of a measuring instrument, such as a questionnaire. It is determined by inspection that the instrument contains important items that measure the variables being studied.
Frequency distribution	The arrangement of the scores or values of characteristics from the highest to the lowest or other systematic way. The distribution of values for a given variable and the number of times each value occurs.
Hawthorne effect	Term used to describe the psychological reactions to the presence of the investigator, or to special treatment during a research study, which tend to alter the responses of the subject. This is often manifested as improvement in the placebo (control) group—the participation effect.
Hypothesis	A statement of predicted relationships between the variables under study; an educated guess by the researcher. It is the testable component of the research. See also *Null hypothesis*.
Independent variable	The variable that is manipulated or changed by the researcher; also called the *manipulated variable;* the presumed cause of change in the dependent variable.

Inductive reasoning	Human reasoning that involves a process in which general rules evolve or develop from individual cases, or observation of phenomena.
Inference	The process by which information gathered from a sample is generalized to a population.
Internal validity	The ability of the research design to answer the research question accurately.
Interrater reliability	Method for determining reliability in which the strength of agreement between the observations made by two or more observers is determined.
Level of significance	The probability level used to reject the null hypothesis (defines how rare or unlikely the sample data must be before the researcher can reject the null hypothesis).
Likert scale	A scale for rating attitudes in which each statement usually has five possible responses: strongly agree, agree, uncertain, disagree, strongly disagree.
Logical positivism	A philosophical school of thought characterized by belief in a singular, knowable reality that exists separate from individual ideas; basis for the scientific method.
Manipulation	Manuevering the independent variable so that the effect of its presence or absence can be observed on the dependent variable(s).
Mean	The arthmetic average; average score.
Measures of central tendency	Numerical information regarding the most typical or representative scores in a group (e.g., mean).
Median	The number above which 50 percent of the observations fall; a measure of central tendency.
MEDLARS	*(Medical Literature Analysis and Retrieval System)* The computerized literature retrieval service of the National Library of Medicine.
MEDLINE	A computerized data base that references biomedical journal articles.
Meta-analysis	The statistical analysis of a large collection of results from several studies for the purpose of integrating the findings into a single, generalized finding.
Mode	The most frequent score in a distribution; the peak (or peaks) in a frequency curve.
Null hypothesis	The most commonly used method of stating the way the relationship between the variables being studied will be tested. The null hypothesis is stated: "There is no statistically significant differ-

ence between the experimental and the control group."

Operational definition — A description that reduces the abstract to a concrete observable form by specifying the exact procedures for measuring or observing a phenomenon.

Phenomenology — Naturalistic inquiry that aims to uncover the meaning of how humans experience phenomena through the description of those experiences as they are lived by individuals.

Primary score — First-hand information obtained from original material; not interpretive or hearsay information; an original article.

Probability value (p value) — A statistical estimate of the likelihood that a finding is due to chance. By convention, a finding with a p value less than 5% (p<.05) is called statistically significant.

Problem statement — A statement that identifies the phenomenon to be explored and why it needs to be examined, or why it is a problem or issue.

Prospective study — A study that begins with presumed causes (e.g., cigarette smoking) and then goes forward in time to observe effects (e.g., lung cancer).

Qualitative data — Data characterized by words (*pale, cyanotic,* etc.).

Quantitative data — Data characterized by numbers.

Quasi-experimental research — Research approach in which the independent variable is manipulated to determine the effect on the dependent variable, but subjects are not randomly assigned to treatment conditions.

Quota sampling — A nonrandom sampling technique in which the investigator purposively obtains a sample by selecting sample elements in the same proportion in which they are represented in the population.

Randomization — Assignment of subjects to treatment conditions in such a manner that each population element has an equal probability of appearing in the sample.

Reliability — The degree to which a measuring instrument obtains consistent results when it is reused.

Replication — Repeating a study using the same study design but different study subjects.

Research — A scientific process of inquiry or experimentation that involves purposeful, systematic, and rigorous collection, analysis, and interpretation of data in order to gain new knowledge or add to the existing body of scientific knowledge.

Research question	A clear query that guides an experimental investigation. The question is concise and narrow and establishes the boundaries or limits as to what concepts, individuals, or phenomena will be examined.
Retrospective studies	Studies that describe and examine phenomena after the fact or after the phenomena have occurred—ex post facto design.
Sample	A smaller part of the target population selected in such a way that the individuals in the study group represent the characteristics of the target population; the subset of the population that participates in the study.
Sampling error	The difference between the values obtained from the sample and those that actually exist in the population.
Selection bias	Preexisting differences between study and control groups; these differences affect the dependent variable in ways that are extraneous to the effect of the independent variable and pose a threat to the internal validty of the study.
Serendipitous finding	Unplanned and unexpected discovery of significant results in a research study not related to the purpose of the study.
Spurious correlations	Correlations that yield high relationship values, but where no relationship actually exists.
Standard deviation	The general indicator of dispersion from the mean; an indicator of the average deviation of scores around the mean.
Statistical power	The probability of rejecting the null hypothesis when it is false or should be rejected.
Statistical significance	The extent to which group differences are a function of chance; by convention, a p value of 5% or less (p<.05).
Target population	The total group of individuals meeting the criteria of interest to the researcher.
Tests of significance	Statistical tests (mathematical procedures) used to determine differences between groups, e.g., the chi-square statistic.
Test-retest reliability	Method for determining reliability in which the same instrument is administered to the same individuals at different times and the two sets of scores are then correlated.
Theory	A set of statements, called *propositions,* that are stated in such a way as to form a logically inter-

	related deductive system; used to summarize existing knowledge and to explain or predict phenomena and their relationships.
Type I error	Rejection of the null hypothesis when it should be accepted; also called the *alpha error;* finding group differences when none exist.
Type II error	Acceptance of the null hypothesis when it should be rejected; also called the *beta error;* failing to find group differences when they exist.
Validity	The extent to which a data-gathering instrument measures what it is supposed to measure.

REFERENCES

1. Abdellah, Faye. *Better Patient Care Through Nursing Research.* New York: Macmillan, 1965 (classic).

2. Abdellah, Faye. *Preparing Nursing Research for the 21st Century.* New York: Springer Publishing, 1994.

3. Beck, Cheryl. "Replication Strategies for Nursing Research." *IMAGE: Journal of Nursing Scholarship* 26(3):191–194, 1994.

4. Beveridge, W. *The Art of Scientific Investigation.* New York: Vintage Books, (Classic). 1957.

5. Borg, Walter. *Educational Research.* New York: Longman, 1989.

6. Brink, Pamela. *Basic Steps to Planning Nursing Research.* Boston: Jones and Bartlett Publishers, 1994.

7. Chauvin, Van. "Clinical Investigations: A Vital Part of School Nurse Practice." *Journal of School Health* 8(3):25–29, 1992.

8. Dempsey, Patricia. *Nursing Research with Basic Statistical Applications.* Boston: Jones and Bartlett, 1992.

9. DePoy, Elizabeth. *Introduction to Research.* St. Louis: Mosby, 1993.

10. Haley, Robert. "Designing Clinical Research." In *Techniques of Patient Oriented Research.* New York: Raven Press, 1994.

11. Hungler, Bernadette. *Study Guide for Nursing Research.* Philadelphia: J. B. Lippincott, 1993.

12. Lang, Thomas. "Why Medical Editors Should Learn About Statistics." *American Medical Writers Association Journal* 9(2):45–50, 1994.

13. Larson, Elaine. "Exclusion of Certain Groups from Clinical Resarch." *IMAGE: Journal of Nursing Scholarship* 26(3):185–190, 1994.

14. Michael, Max. *Biomedical Bestiary: An Epidemiologic Guide to Flaws and Fallacies in the Medical Literature.* Boston: Little Brown, 1984.

15. Morton, Richard. *A Study Guide to Epidemiology and Biostatistics.* Gaithersburg, MD: Aspen Publications, 1989.

16. Polit, Denise. *Essentials of Nursing Research.* Philadelphia: J. B. Lippincott, 1993.

17. Polit, Denise, and B. Hungler. *Study Guide for Nursing Research.* Philadelphia: J. B. Lippincott, 1991.

18. Riegelman, Richard. *Studying a Study and Testing a Test.* Boston: Little Brown, 1989.

19. Rimm, A. *Basic Biostatistics in Medicine and Epidemiology.* New York: Appleton-Century-Crofts, 1980.

20. Rowntree, D. *Statistics Without Tears.* New York: Charles Scribner's Sons, 1981.

21. Sumner, D. Lies, Damned Lies—or Statistics?" *Journal of Hypertension* 10(1):306, 1992.

22. Vaughan, Roger. "The Role of the Medical Communicator in Preventing Disease." *American Medical Writers Association Journal* 9(2):39–42, 1994.

Figure 11-1

PRIORITIES FOR NURSING RESEARCH*

1. Promote the ability to care for oneself.

2. Minimize or prevent behaviorally and environmentally induced health problems.

3. Ensure that the health care needs of vulnerable groups are met in effective and acceptable ways.

4. Classify nursing practice phenomena.

5. Develop instruments to measure nursing outcomes.

6. Develop methodologies for the study of human beings as they relate to their families and lifestyles.

7. Evaluate alternative models for delivering health care and for administering health care systems so that nurses will be able to balance high quality with cost-effectiveness.

8. Evaluate the effectiveness of alternative approaches to nursing education.

9. Ensure that ethical principles guide nursing research.

*Modified from Polit (1993).

Figure 11-2

VARIABLES IN RESEARCH*

Dependent Variables

    Also called: outcome variables
                            response variables
                            effect variables

Independent Variables

    Also called: treatment variables
                            causal variables
                            risk factors

Extraneous Variables

    Also called: confounding variables
                            biasing variables
                            co-variables

*Modified from Haley (1994).

Figure 11-3

CONTINUUM OF EXPERIMENTAL DESIGN

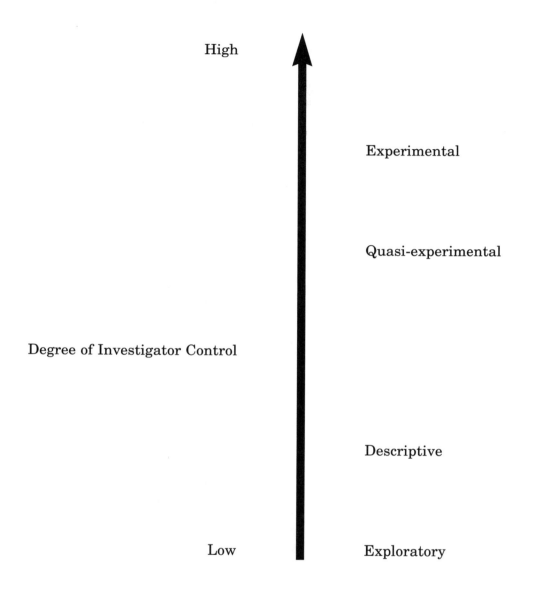

Figure 11-4

SEQUENCE OF EXPERIMENTAL RESEARCH

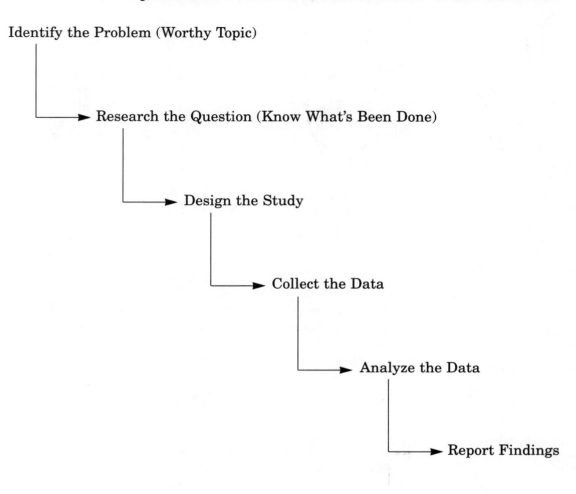

Identify the Problem (Worthy Topic)

Research the Question (Know What's Been Done)

Design the Study

Collect the Data

Analyze the Data

Report Findings

Figure 11-5

LEVELS IN THE SAMPLING PROCESS

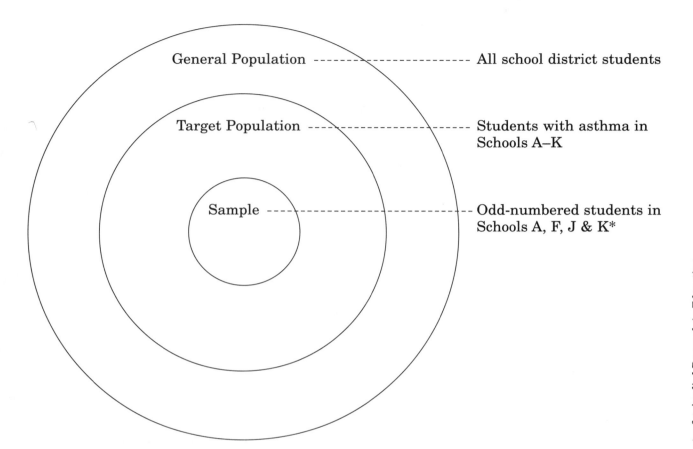

General Population -------------------------- All school district students

Target Population ---------------------- Students with asthma in
Schools A–K

Sample ------------------------ Odd-numbered students in
Schools A, F, J & K*

*From alphabetical list of enrollees.

Figure 11-6

SUMMARY FORM FOR A RESEARCH PROTOCOL

Investigator: Date:

Title:

I.   Statement of Problem

II. Summary of Literature Review

III. Statement of Purpose of the Study

IV. Operational Definitions of Terms (attach additional pages, if necessary)

V.   Data Collection Plan (include instruments to be used)

VI. Plan for Data Analysis

Figure 11-7

DATA COLLECTION APPROACHES IN
SELF-REPORT STUDIES

- Structured personal interviews

- Distributed questionnaires

- Mailed questionnaires

- Structured telephone interviews

- Unstructured personal interviews

- Focus group interviews

Figure 11-8

QUESTIONNAIRE VS. INTERVIEW

QUESTIONNAIRE ADVANTAGES	INTERVIEW ADVANTAGES
1. Less expensive.	1. Higher response rate of subjects.
2. Subjects feel more anonymous.	2. Questions may be explained if not understood.
3. Format standard for all subjects.	3. Data gathered is not limited by predetermined questions.
4. Large samples, covering large geographic areas can be taken.	4. Subject need not be able to read or write.
5. Greater amount of data can be collected.	5. Interviewer can observe subjects' responses.

Figure 11-9

SOME TYPES OF ERRORS IN RESEARCH

ACTIVITY	ERROR
1. research questions operational definitions	1. lack of face validity
2. development of measurement instrument (quesitonnaire)	2. ambiguous wording of questions; categories not mutually exclusive
3. subject selection	3. sampling error (not representative)
4. data collection	4. reliability issues (mood of subject; faulty recording, etc.)
5. data analysis	5. wrong statistical method chosen; faulty interpretation

Figure 11-10

JOURNAL OF SCHOOL NURSING
GUIDELINES FOR AUTHORS

What is the *Journal of School Nursing's* purpose?

The major purpose of the *Journal of School Nursing* is to provide a forum for promoting the professional growth of school nurses and advancing the practice of school nursing. Original clinical, nonclinical, and research articles on topics of interest or importance to school nurses are sought by the journal.

Form

Manuscripts should be typed, double-spaced, on one side of 8 1/2 x 11 inch white paper, maximum length, 14 pages (3,500 words). A cover sheet should include title of the manuscript, author(s) name(s), credentials and primary affiliations, and address and telephone numbers (work and home) of the primary author. Acknowledgement of foundation and grant support, if any, also needs to be noted. This page should be followed by an abstract of approximately 50 words. The manuscript title should be repeated on the first page of the text. Author(s) name(s) should not appear elsewhere on the manuscript.

Style

The third edition of the *American Psychological Association Publication Manual* (1983) provides the format for references, photographs, tables, and other details. References in the text should be cited by author and date, for example, (Smith & Jones, 1987), with page numbers cited for direct quotations. Tables should be typed, double-spaced, one to a page, titled, and relative placement in the text noted. Figures and diagrams should include title, typed on a separate page. Color slides need to be clearly labeled (top, bottom, right, left) and placement in the text noted. Authors are responsible for obtaining written permission to reproduce any material with preexisting copyright.

Procedure

Query letters to the Editor are welcomed but not required. Manuscripts are received with the assurance that they are not simultaneously under consideration by any other publication. Receipt of manuscript is acknowledged by the Editor. The *Journal of School Nursing* is a refereed journal. Manuscripts are reviewed (without author identification) by at least three reviewers from the Manuscript Review Panel, and decisions for publication are made on the basis of the reviews. Revision is sometimes necessary. Accepted manuscripts become the property of the *Journal of School Nursing*. Manuscripts not accepted for publication will not be returned to the authors. The *Journal of School Nursing* reserves the right to edit all manuscripts to its style and space requirements and to clarify the presentation. Authors will receive proofs for approval and assume final responsibility for content of the manuscript, including the edited copy.

Four copies of the manuscript will be sent to Editor, *Journal of School Nursing,* Yale University School of Nursing, 25 Park Street, P. O. Box 9740, New Haven, CT 06536-0740.

Figure 11-11

SCHEDULE FOR A RESEARCH PROJECT

July	Literature Review
August	Design Protocol & Select Subjects (Seek funding source if appropriate)
September	
October	Implement Study
November	&
December	Collect Data
January	Analyze Data
February	Write-up of Study
March	Submit for Publication

CHAPTER 12

LEGAL FRAMEWORKS FOR SCHOOL HEALTH

LEGAL FRAMEWORKS FOR SCHOOL HEALTH

> The public is not always sagacious, but in the long run, it does somehow contrive to find out who are the skilled lawyers.
>
> *John Shaw Billings (1838–1913)*

If you are one of those people who considers legal issues mystical and anxiety producing, you are not alone. Concern over legal liability is one of the most frequently discussed topics in nursing circles—not surprising in light of our increasingly litigious society. The theoretical risk looms large; however, in practice there are surprisingly few lawsuits against school nurses. Knowing your profession and the legal framework in which you practice is the best defense against actual suits and "paralysis legalis"—failure to act due to fear of legal liability. You do not want to withhold a clear benefit from a student because of a theoretical legal risk.

A simple definition of law is: a body of official rules and regulations found in constitutions, legislation, and judicial opinions that are used to govern a society and to control the behavior of its members. The law is backed by the coercive power of the state (federal, state, and local governments), which enforces it through penalties. Laws limiting the powers of government help to provide a degree of individual freedom. Law is also used as a mechanism for social change, for instance, to inhibit social discrimination and to improve the quality of individual life in matters of health, education, and welfare.

HOW THE FEDERAL GOVERNMENT AFFECTS SCHOOLS

The U.S. Constitution

Most of our basic civil liberties are included in the Bill of Rights (first ten amendments to the Constitution). The First Amendment is particularly important. It lists several liberties inherent in a domestic society: the right to be free from government control in the exercise of speech, publication, religious preference, and assembly. However, the First Amendment, like the other nine, applies only to the federal government.

To discover what U.S. Constitutional rights we enjoy in the state setting, we must look to the Fourteenth Amendment: "nor shall any State deprive any person of life, liberty, or property without due process of law, nor deny any person within its jurisdiction the equal protection of the laws." This clause provides the basis for constitutional rights suits against public educational institutions and personnel: due process, and equal protection. Local public school districts are viewed as state political subdivisions. The Fourteenth Amendment does not apply to private schools.

Neither liberty rights nor property rights are without limits. They can be regulated, even denied, provided the state or school follows due process—a proceeding, usually in a court of law, where a person is served with notice and has an opportunity to be heard and protect her or his rights.

Behavior that is not constitutionally protected as a liberty or property right can be regulated relatively easily. Smoking and the possession of hallucinogenic drugs fall into this category.

The fact that the U.S. Constitution does not protect certain types of behavior does not mean that a state legislature or school district cannot decide to do so. For example, some school districts grant students personal grooming rights, though they may legally establish a dress code.

Important Federal Laws

- *Title VI of the Civil Rights Act (1964)*: prohibits institutional discrimination on the basis of race, color, or national origin in federally assisted programs.

- *Title VII of the Civil Rights Act*: prohibits discrimination on the basis of race, color, religion, sex, or national origin in all aspects of public and private employment.

- *Americans with Disabilities Act (1990)*: accords persons with disabilities meaningful access to programs and facilities of public schools, as well as most businesses. It requires employers to make "reasonable accommodation" for disabled persons to enable them to perform the job.

- *Title IX of the Education Amendments (1972)*: prohibits discrimination on the basis of sex in any federally assisted education program. Title IX has gained major significance in the context of student and employee sexual harassment.

- *Individuals with Disabilities Education Act (IDEA)*: requires public schools to identify children with disabilities and provide a free and appropriate public education in the least restrictive environment.

- *Goals 2000: Educate America Act (P.L. 103–227)(1994)*: codified several national education goals and authorized funds for K–12 school improvement. The goals focus on (1) improving student learning by establishing objectives for students and schools, (2) encouraging states and local school districts to adopt rigorous standards, (3) improving the quality of teaching K–12, and (4) identifying common standards for student achievement.

FEDERAL LAW ADDRESSING STUDENT RIGHTS

Student Records and Privacy

By the very nature of the educational process, educators are constantly dealing in sensitive matters involving students' private and personal affairs. Schools routinely collect and process information about students that can materially affect their future lives. Personal information that is carelessly released may well attach a stigma to a student's image in the community or establish an educational black mark that detracts from the student's success in future educational and business pursuits.

The law protects the student in three ways. First, school districts are required to handle and process student records in a careful and prescribed manner by federal statute; failure to do so can result in the loss of federal funds. A number of states also have statutes mandating procedures for protecting the student's right of privacy. Second, the law allows the student protection through court precedents that form the law of defamation (case law). Third, the student has a right of privacy protected by the common law right against invasion of privacy.

The Family Educational Rights and Privacy Act of 1974, more popularly known as the Buckley Amendment, prescribes standards for schools to follow in handling student records. Parents are given the right to inspect all records that schools maintain on their children and the opportunity to challenge the accuracy of the records. Parents must consent before the school can release the student's records to agencies outside designated educational categories. Consent may also be given by the student, in lieu of the parent, to release his or her own records when the student reaches eighteen or enters college. School districts that do not follow the procedures required risk losing federal funds administered by the United States Department of Education. See more on the Buckley Amendment under Parents' Rights.

Defamation

Anyone—teacher, administrator, parent, or student—is capable of incurring liability by defaming other persons. Words are defamatory if they impute to another dishonesty, immorality, vice or dishonorable conduct that creates a negative opinion of the person in the minds of others in a community. Defamation is anything that tends to injure one's character or reputation.

The distinction between *criticism* and *defamation* is that criticism is addressed to public matters and does not follow a person into his or her private life. A true critic never indulges in personal ridicule but confines his or her comments to the merits of the particular subject matter under discussion.

Defamation is not a legal cause of action but encompasses the twin liabilities of *libel* and *slander*. Libel is written defamation while slander is spoken.

Progress notes, carelessly written by a school nurse, can be the basis for a libel suit: "This student is apparently promiscuous." The best safeguard is to limit entries to objective observations. Opinions and judgments have no place in student progress notes.

Courts have found it necessary to extend limited privileges to certain persons in society where the public interest requires such protection. Such *conditional* or *qualified* privileges are extended to teachers and school administrators as well as to other public servants who are charged with duties requiring them to handle sensitive information. The rationale for such protection is: "In order that the information may be freely given, it is necessary to afford protection against liability for misinformation given in an appropriate effort to protect or advance the interest in question." If protection were not given, information that should be given or received would not be communicated because of fear of liability.

The degree of protection afforded by the conditional or qualified privilege is determined by the courts in weighing "on one hand, society's need for free disclosure without fear of civil suit, and on the other hand, an individual's right to recover for damage to his or her reputation."

The conditional privilege negates any presumption of implied malice from the defamatory statement, and places the burden on the plaintiff to show proof of actual malice. One can easily see that teachers and nurses would be hesitant to convey any information at all about students if no privilege existed. Without such conditional privilege, reports both academic and disciplinary would hold great potential for legal actions.

In order for the privilege of the teacher or administrator to withstand challenge, the communication must have been made (1) in good faith, without malice, and within the scope of the student's, teacher's, or public's interest; (2) in the honest belief that the information conveyed was true, with knowledge that any communication brought about a student was made on reasonable grounds; and (3) in response to a legitimate inquiry by one with the right to know about a student's educational or personal qualification and that the answer does not go beyond that required to satisfy the inquiry. Volunteering excessive information not bearing on the student's or the school's interests is hazardous.

Freedom of Association

High school students have a right to assemble peacefully for expressive purposes in the vicinity of the public school. The support given the right of association, coupled with the recognition of student free speech rights, indicates that students at the secondary level also have a right to come together for expressive purposes on the public school campus as long as no disruption or invasion of the rights of others occurs. Because the public school is not a public forum, however, the right of association does not automatically extend to nonstudents.

Does the right to associate restrict school officials in deciding which student groups may and which may not function as school-recognized organizations? The answer depends on the type of group and the legitimacy of the school's reasons in denying status as a campus organization to a student group. For example, a federal district court in Michigan ruled in the early 1970s that it is unconstitutional to deny recognition in the absence of disorder to student groups because they advocate controversial ideas or take one side of an issue. Most state laws explicitly prohibit the existence of fraternities, sororities, and secret societies in public elementary and secondary schools. Some school districts are using these provisions to bar gangs from school premises.

There are other student organizations, however, that fall in a gray area. What about controversial organizations, such as a student gay rights group or a religious organization? Should they be accorded official recognition as student clubs if they obtain a faculty sponsor and meet other criteria for school recognition? The answer remains unclear. In some cases, school officials may seek to refuse recognition on grounds that the existence of such a school-sanctioned organization would have a detrimental impact on younger students. In the case of an extremist group, the school might argue that its presence would be likely to trigger disruption.

The U.S. Supreme Court has not yet dealt directly with student organizations; however, in a 1989 decision, the Court ruled that the right of association protected by the First Amendment relates to expressive activities and not to those that are strictly social. Local school boards set the policy, but it may be challenged unless all student groups are judged by the same criteria.

Search and Seizure

To search or not to search a pupil's desk, locker, pockets, or purse, is a question frequently confronting school administrations. Many times the issue must be decided quickly due to the seriousness of a situation—bomb threats, dangerous weapons, illegal drugs—that could result in injury.

Students have a right of privacy—to be secure in their persons, papers, and effects—and this right protects them against unreasonable searches and seizures. Any search must be specific as to what is sought and the location. The courts do not require school officials to provide evidence of "probable cause" or to obtain a warrant justifying a search from a judge.

Avoid involvement in searches of a student's person, as your participation undermines your established helping role and places you in a disciplinary role.

Truancy

The federal government is silent on the matter of truancy and leaves each state to establish its own standards. The states hold parents accountable and many assess stiff fines for nonattendance up to a certain age, usually 16. See the section on parents' rights in this chapter.

Students with Disabilities: IDEA

No area of school law has experienced such explosive growth over the past 15 years as that of special education. Since the mid-1970s, the rights of students with disabilities have been increasingly subject to legislation and litigation. School nurses are intimately involved in identifying and serving children with disabilities.

Some of the important regulations and acronyms of special education are:

- *P.L. 94-142*: The landmark legislation passed by Congress in 1975 guaranteeing every child with a disability a free, appropriate public education. Known as the Education for All Handicapped Children Act, it has now been expanded and renamed IDEA.

- *IDEA*: Individuals with Disabilities Education Act (1990).

- *504*: Section 504 of the 1973 Rehabilitation Act—a federal law prohibiting discrimination against persons with disabilities in programs that receive federal funds.

- *FAPE*: Free, Appropriate Public Education. The law mandates that FAPE be available to every child, regardless of the nature or severity of the disability.

- *IEP*: Individual Education Plan. This is the written planning tool for the child's education. It is collaboratively developed by school officials and parents.

- *LRC*: Local Review Committee—the local school group that first reviews a child's need and eligibility for special education and related services.

- *Related Services*: Special transportation and other noninstructional services that are necessary for the child to obtain benefit from the educational program. These also include occupational therapy, physical therapy, speech therapy, counseling, and other services.

- *Placement*: The instructional arrangement in which the child is educated. It can range from the regular classroom to a special residential school.

  - *LRE*: Least Restrictive Environment. The placement of the child must be in the LRE that is appropriate. It must enable the child to interact with his or her peers who are not disabled to the extent possible, given the nature and severity of the disability.

- *Handicapping Condition*: To be eligible for federally funded special education services, the child must meet eligibility criteria for one of several categories. These include learning disabled (LD), emotionally disturbed (ED), mentally retarded (MR), other health impaired (OHI), visually handicapped (VH), and auditorially handicapped (AH).

It is difficult to conceive of a piece of legislation with better intentions than IDEA. The steps to be followed are: identification, assessment, LRC, IEP, and placement. Schools are required to take affirmative action to make sure every eligible child in the district is identified and evaluated. Referrals can be made by parents, teachers, doctors, psychologists, or others familiar with the child.

Assessment procedures must guarantee that children are assessed in their native language, that measurement instruments are not racially or culturally biased, that tests are validated for the specific purpose for which they are used, that tests are administered by trained personnel in accordance with their instructions, and that no single criterion (e.g., IQ score) is used to determine an appropriate program for the child. Parents who disagree with the school's assessment of their child have the right to obtain an independent educational evaluation.

Members of the LRC are expected to work collaboratively to develop a program for each child. When they do so and are able to reach a consensus, few legal issues arise.

The singular principle that applies to special education law is the concept of individualized decision making. The IEP is a written statement of services to be delivered and goals to be achieved. The law requires that the IEP include

- educational achievement levels
- annual goals with short-term objectives
- special education and related services to be provided (including the extent to which the child will participate in a regular education program)
- dates when services are to begin and expected duration of services
- objective criteria and evaluation procedures for determining progress

The law requires that each school district have a system for parents to challenge decisions regarding their child in a due process hearing, before going to court.

The area of "related services" may involve you. The definitions of "medical services" and "school health services" are crucial in knowing what schools must provide. The courts have taken the position that "medical services," which a school district is not required to provide, are those that must be delivered by a physician or a hospital. The only medical services required of a school district are those for diagnostic or evaluative purposes. In the Irving ISD vs. Tatro case regarding bladder catheterizing at school, the Supreme Court noted that school nurses typically provide a variety of services for children and that clean intermittent catheterization (CIC) could be accomplished by a school nurse or even a layperson.

In drawing the distinction between medical services and related services, the courts look at four factors:

- Is the service constant or periodic?
- Does the service require a health care professional?
- Is the service complex or simple?
- Is the service economically reasonable?

The Tatro case was successful because the service was periodic, did not require a health professional, and was simple and inexpensive. Cases where students have sought the constant attention of a nurse to perform a variety of complex procedures at considerable expense to the school have been unsuccessful.

Section 504

The definition of "handicapping condition" in Section 504 is broader than in IDEA: a handicapped student is one who has a physical or mental impairment that substantially limits one or more life activities (working, eating, dressing, breathing, learning, etc.). The Office of Civil Rights, which oversees enforcement of the statute, has determined that this may include drug and alcohol addiction, attention deficit disorder, AIDS, hospitalization due to depression, and other conditions not included under IDEA. IDEA funds cannot be used to comply with 504.

School districts are just now beginning to deal with the implications of 504 for students not eligible under IDEA.

FEDERAL LAW ADDRESSING PARENTS' RIGHTS AND RESPONSIBILITIES

Minors vs. Majority-Age Students

Parents are the agents for their minor children (under 18) and are thus responsible for monitoring and challenging the implementation of all student rights as outlined above. Parents must give consent for most services rendered in schools. Even those services mandated by state law (e.g., vision and hearing screening, immunizations) are subject to certain exemptions upon parent request: for example, religious exemption from immunization. Students 18 years and older may make decisions for themselves.

Buckley Amendment

The Buckley Amendment, referred to in the section on student rights, allows parents access to virtually all school records relating to their child. They have the right to appeal anything in a student's file that is considered incorrect, and if the school is not willing to delete the challenged material, to request a hearing.

Exemptions to Parental Consent

Parental consent is not required for release of education records (1) to other school officials or teachers in the school system who have legitimate educational interests; (2) to officials of other schools or school systems in which the student seeks to enroll, upon the condition that the student's parents are notified of the transfer of records, and have an opportunity to challenge the record; (3) to authorized representatives of government, including state education authorities; (4) in connection with a student's application for financial aid; (5) to state and local officials collecting information required by state statutes adopted before November 19, 1974; (6) to organizations conducting studies for, or on behalf of, educational agencies if personal identification of students is destroyed when no longer needed for the study; (7) to accrediting organizations; or (8) in compliance with regulations of the Secretary of Education pertaining to health or welfare of the student or other persons.

Beyond these exceptions, no personally identifiable information can be released, other than directory information, without written consent of the parent specifying the records to be released. Schools must, of course, respond to subpoenas issued by the courts for information but must notify parents of such occurrences.

Personal Notes

Personal notes (such as a school nurse might keep but not record on any official record) are considered "not education records" and are exempted from parental access. Personal notes that are not accessible to other school staff are also exempted from student or parental access.

Competency Challenges

Parents have a qualified privilege to speak publicly before a school board regarding a teacher's instruction of their children or the performance of any other professional employee of the school district, including the school nurse. It is within the right of parents to oversee their children's education—to make statements pertaining to a teacher's (or other school professional's) efficiency and competency. The burden of proving incompetency or malice rests with the parent (plaintiff).

Truancy

Compulsory attendance laws provide for enforcement by penalizing parents for their children's absences. When a child is declared a chronic truant, the school board may institute legal proceedings that may include criminal penalty for the parent. A typical definition of truant is: "a child subject to compulsory school attendance who is absent without valid excuse from such attendance for one or more school days."

Valid causes for absences may be variously defined by state statutes as illness: death in the family, family emergency, or situations beyond the control of the student. A physician statement may be required.

FEDERAL LAW GOVERNING SCHOOL EMPLOYEES

Education is a state responsibility; consequently, little specific federal legislation exists in this area, with the exception of special education, which dictates certain professional activities. School employees are, of course, entitled to all the generic rights and privileges guaranteed under the Constitution.

The assurance of teacher competency was, to some degree, a response to compulsory attendance. If the state compelled children to attend school, then these children should be supervised and taught by qualified or certified teachers and other professionals. Certification differs in each state depending on the statutory provisions and regulations. Each state has the responsibility for certification or decertification (revocation of license) and usually this responsibility is delegated to the State Board of Education.

Chapter 8 covers the health and disability issues for school employees contained in the Americans with Disabilities Act and Section 504 of the Rehabilitation Act. The main issues center around preemployment inquiries and on-the-job accommodations for disabled individuals.

Most states provide a degree of immunity from legal liability to school employees by virtue of the fact that school districts are an extension of the state government. In most states school employees cannot be sued in the course of their regular duties short of assaults or "gross negligence."

STATE GOVERNANCE OF PUBLIC SCHOOLS

State government, through statute, regulates and controls education subject only to limitations placed on it by the state and federal constitutions. The courts have consistently held that the power over education is an essential attribute of state sovereignty of the same order as the power to tax, to exercise police power, and to provide for the welfare of the citizens. In the exercise of this function, states have established systems of public schools that are operated as administrative arms of the state government.

In holding that education is a state function, the courts maintain that the state's authority over education is not a distributive one, to be exercised by local government, but is a central power residing in the state. The legislature has the prerogative to prescribe the methods of education, and the courts will not intervene unless the legislation is contrary to constitutional provisions.

State legislatures may delegate powers to local school districts, usually through a chief state school officer who is often called the State Commissioner of Education. It is well established, then, that the local school district is a state agency that operates at a local level.

Because local school boards are state bodies, it follows that school board members are state, not local, officials. Local school boards are vested with a portion of the sovereignty of the state through delegation, by which they acquire certain administrative functions having characteristics of all three branches of government: executive, legislative, and judicial. Their policies have the force of law.

In challenging the exercise of administrative powers by an educational agency, the aggrieved parties are required to exhaust their administrative remedies before they are allowed to bring an action before the courts. Such a rule assures the courts that issues have been properly treated at lower levels, thus preventing continuous involvement of the courts in educational disputes where legitimate legal controversy is not present.

SCHOOL NURSES AND THE LAW

It would be ideal if school nurses could devote 100% of their energies toward providing quality health care to their clients. They are good at it, and they enjoy what they do. But the litigation explosion has forced school nurses not only to keep abreast of professional knowledge, but to become aware of the risks of legal liability. Fortunately, few school nurses have been personally named in lawsuits. Perhaps that is because they have been proactive in learning the legal implications of their practice.

Health vs. Education Law

The convergence of health and education law is diagrammed in Figure 12-1, at the end of this chapter. You and your supervisors may often be required to interpret and resolve existing conflict by deciding which takes precedence—health or education law. School attorneys are the experts in this area.

When school nurses ask, "Is it legal?" what they mean is, "Will I go to court?" In examining any given issue, you and your legal consultant will want to review applicable federal and state statutes as well as case law. The latter is made up of the decisions in previous court cases. In some subject areas, the laws are silent and case law is the only guide. Keep in mind that state education and health department regulations have the force of law and, if in conflict, may require a state attorney general's opinion to resolve the issue. Figure 12-2 tabulates some sources of legal guidelines.

Types of Liability

Three kinds of legal liability exist:

- criminal
- civil
- professional regulatory

Diverting a student's Ritalin for illicit use by others is an example of criminal liability. Most cases fall in the civil liability category and involve personal injury to the client. The third category, professional regulatory liability, usually involves breech of the state nurse practice act or unethical actions that may result in suspension of licensure.

In civil liability four proofs are required for a successful case:

- A duty or obligation exists.
- A breech of that duty occurred.
- The breech caused injury.
- Actual damage is demonstrated.

There is no case if no injury occurred, even if a negligent act was committed.

The criteria for "duty or obligation" hinges on the accepted standard of care (SOC). Documents that make up the SOC include the nurse's job description, national standards (e.g., ANA Standards of Clinical Nursing Practice), and, of course, state law, as well as state board of education and health department guidelines. Expert witnesses are often used to establish community practice norms. The legal test applied is, "What would a reasonable and prudent nurse have done in a similar situation?"

Key Liability Issues

Nadine Schwab (see references), a prominent national voice on the liability issues facing school nurses, has identified the three issues of greatest concern:

- delegation
- confidentiality
- do not resuscitate (DNR) orders

In her 1994 presentation at the National Association of School Nurses Annual meeting, she identified five potential causes of legal confusion:

- conflicts between health and education law
- conflicts between nursing standards of care and school district policies

- lack of clarity in the law regarding nursing practice in school settings
- lack of supervision and clinical support for school nurses
- civil rights of individuals with disabilities versus nursing standards

Causes of Nursing Liability

Some recurring causes of nursing liability include:

- ignorance of current professional knowledge and practice
- inadequate health history
- inadequate assessment
- failure to observe and report (or act on) changes in client's status
- failure to document properly
- failure to report incompetent care by others
- failure to carry out physician orders
- failure to challenge improper physician orders
- improper aseptic technique
- abandonment
- failure to resuscitate promptly

One of your most important acts is adequate documentation. To gain perspective on what is adequate, imagine each of your health record entries as "exhibit A" in a court room: Is it detailed enough and objective enough to show that you acted appropriately? Does it avoid libelous opinons and judgments? There is no case if the client contributed to his or her own harm through negligence, so documentation of recommendations to students and parents is especially important.

School nurses are fortunate in that they are less likely to incur legal liability than their colleagues in hospitals; they benefit from a degree of sovereign immunity by virtue of the fact that public school districts are an arm of state government. Assault and gross negligence are not included in this immunity.

Delegation

Although delegation to unlicensed persons, such as nurse's aides, is a valid concern, it has been my experience that school nurses are quite careful and conscientious in this regard. Three key elements of appropriate delegation are

- written instructions
- documentation of completed training
- ongoing monitoring

Complex tasks requiring nursing judgment should never be delegated. Know what your state board of nurse examiners says about specific tasks that may be delegated.

Confidentiality

School nurses have an excellent track record in this area. Contrast this with the gossip about student problems heard in teachers' lounges. There are times, however, when confidentiality should not be maintained.

- written consent of parents obtained
- internal communication to a professional colleague
- medical or psychiatric emergency (e.g., suicide threat)
- court order
- a crime has been, or is about to be, committed
- required audit
- child abuse

It should be obvious that lists of students and their medical diagnoses should not be circulated in the school. Communicate with teachers in a student-specific and private way.

"Do Not Resuscitate" Orders

Some school attorneys have advised nurses in schools never to honor DNR orders. This is a rigid opinion that can lead to potential liability for assault and battery if the nurse institutes CPR against the written, legal request of the parent and valid order of a physician. Case-by-case planning is the best course of action. Should you elect to honor a DNR order, the county medical examiner's (coroner's) office and local emergency medical service should be notified. A field agent from the coroner's office can pronounce death in most states and a funeral home may pick up the body directly from the school (in an unmarked vehicle, of course)—no sirens or fanfare. If death is inevitable, then dignity is the primary concern. The student's wishes must of course be considered when the age of majority is reached.

Duty to Client

An important guiding principle is: Who is the client? It is always the student (and parents)—never the employer. You must always differentiate between duty to your employer and duty to your client and nursing ethics—a juggling act requiring sound judgment. The courts continue to clarify duty issues, but will never be able to give you a definitive answer for every possible scenario.

Documentation

NASN has identified five areas requiring documentation:

- data base/assessment information
- nursing diagnoses and collaborative health problems
- planning
- implementation of care
- evaluation of care

Clinical documentation of school nursing services includes the written notes and records of nursing care provided to an individual student. Clinical documentation needs will vary depending on the population of students served, the types of health services provided in the school district, and staffing patterns. In any setting, however, you must develop documentation practices that are in keeping with the nursing process. The time-honored legal axiom applies here: *If it isn't written down, it didn't happen.*

The student health record is the primary format for documentation of your activities. Figure 12-3 is an example of a comprehensive student health record, with space for progress notes. Note that a portion (demographic data, screening, and immunization results) may be copied and sent to another school without signed parent permission. Another important record is the Individualized Health Care Plan (Chapter 2), used for students with complex medical problems and those enrolled in special education.

Strategies for Avoiding Liability

Linda S. Gilman, past president of NAPNAP (National Association of Pediatric Nurse Associates and Practitioners) recommends the following steps to minimize the risk of legal liability (see references):

- Know your state's Nurse Practice Act.
- Communicate with your clients.
- Use *Standards of School Nursing Practice* (ANA) as a guide.
- Keep your knowledge base up-to-date.
- Don't allow yourself to be placed in situations you are not prepared to handle.
- Clearly document your findings.
- Make timely and appropriate referrals.
- Develop practice protocols.
- Have a peer review system in place.

In addition to this list: Ensure that your job description is current, and get to know your school attorney or other legal advisor.

Ethics

Broadly defined, *ethics* encompasses moral duty and obligation. Most professionals have a formalized system of values. Key elements of the NASN Code of Ethics include

1. Client Care

   The school nurse is an advocate for students, families, and members of the school community. The school nurse provides health services, while recognizing each individual's inherent right to be treated with dignity and confidentiality, and works to support the client's active participation in health decisions.

2. Professional Competency

   The school nurse maintains the highest level of competency by enhancing professional knowledge and skills, and by collaborating with peers, other health professionals and community agencies, adhering to the Standards of School Nursing Practice.

3. Professional Responsibilities

   The school nurse participates in the profession's efforts to advance the standards of practice, expand the body of knowledge through nursing research, and improve conditions of employment.

The NASN resolutions in Figures 12-4 and 12-5 further define this organization's ethical standards: Human and Civil Rights for Students, and Human and Civil Rights for School Nurses.

SUMMARY

Your best protection against legal liability lies in staying professionally current, focusing on the client, practicing within the framework of the law, and documenting actions and recommendations. Errors of omission take the most effort to avoid (failure to take an adequate history, failure to observe, etc.), but good faith intent goes a long way in court—as does your knowledge of standards of practice and professional ethics.

REFERENCES

1. Alexander, Kern. *American Public School Law.* St. Paul: West Publishing, 1992.

2. ———. *The Law of Schools, Students, and Teachers in a Nutshell.* St. Paul: West Publishing, 1984.

3. Bjorklun, Eugene. "Show and Tell: The Establishment of Religion, and Freedom of Speech." *West's Education Law Quarterly* 3(1):1–10, 1994. (Advises teachers that parents who send their children to public schools have the right to expect instruction that is free from religious indoctrination.)

4. Black, Henry. *Black's Law Dictionary.* St. Paul: West Publishing, 1979.

5. *Code of Ethics.* Scarborough, ME: National Association of School Nurses, 1990.

6. Crawford, Cathlene. "Relief Is Just a Motion Away." *Teaching Exceptional Children* 26(2):26–29, 1994. (Considers legal aspects of conflicts for schools wishing to exclude a child perceived as dangerous in the context of procedural safeguards of the Individuals with Disabilities Education Act.)

7. Dalton, Harlon (ed.). *AIDS and the Law.* New Haven: Yale University Press, 1987.

8. Drager, Elaine. "Impartiality Under the Individuals with Disabilities Education Act." *West's Education Law Quarterly* 3(1):180–209, 1994.

9. Earley, Penelope. *Goals 2000: Educate America Act: Implications for Teacher Educators.* Washington, DC: AACTE Publications, 1994.

10. Gelfman, Mary. "School Health Services and Educational Records: Conflicts in the Law." *Education Law Report,* No. 319, January 31, 1991.

11. Gilman, Linda. "Minimizing Risk of Liability." *Journal of Pediatric Health Care* 1(5):270, 1987.

12. *Guidelines for School Nursing Documentation: Standards, Issues, and Models.* Scarborough, ME: National Association of School Nurses, 1991.

13. Kemerer, Frank. "How the U.S. Constitution and Federal Government Affect Schools." In *The Educators Guide to Texas School Law,* pp. 18–22. Austin: University of Texas Press, 1994.

14. Proctor, S. *School Nursing Practice: Roles and Standards.* Scarborough, ME: National Association of School Nurses, 1993.

15. *Resolutions and Policy Statements.* Scarborough, ME: National Association of School Nurses, 1990.

16. Rose, Deborah. *Providing Public Education Services to Young Children with Disabilities in Community-Based Programs.* Washington, DC: U.S. Department of Education, 1994. (Three federal laws are reviewed: IDEA, the Head Start Act, and the Americans with Disabilities Act [ADA].)

17. "School Nurses and the Law." *Community Nurse Forum* 5(1):1–8, 1988.

18. Schwab, Nadine. "Liability Issues Facing the School Nurse" (audiotape, 2 vols.) Scarborough, ME: National Association of School Nurses, 1994.

19. ———. "School Health Records: Nursing Practice and the Law." *School Nurse* 7(2):17–21, 1991.

20. Snyder, Alicia (ed.). *Implementation Guide for the Standards of School Nursing Practice.* Kent, OH: American School Health Association, 1991.

21. *Standards of School Nurse Practice.* Kansas City, MO: American Nurse's Association, 1983.

22. *Statement on Nursing Care in Schools.* Chicago: National Council of State Boards of Nursing, 1991.

23. Zirkel, Perry. "Section 504: The New Generation of Special Education Cases." *West's Education Law Quarterly* 3(1):128–46, 1994.

Figure 12-1

CONVERGENCE OF EDUCATION AND HEALTH LAW

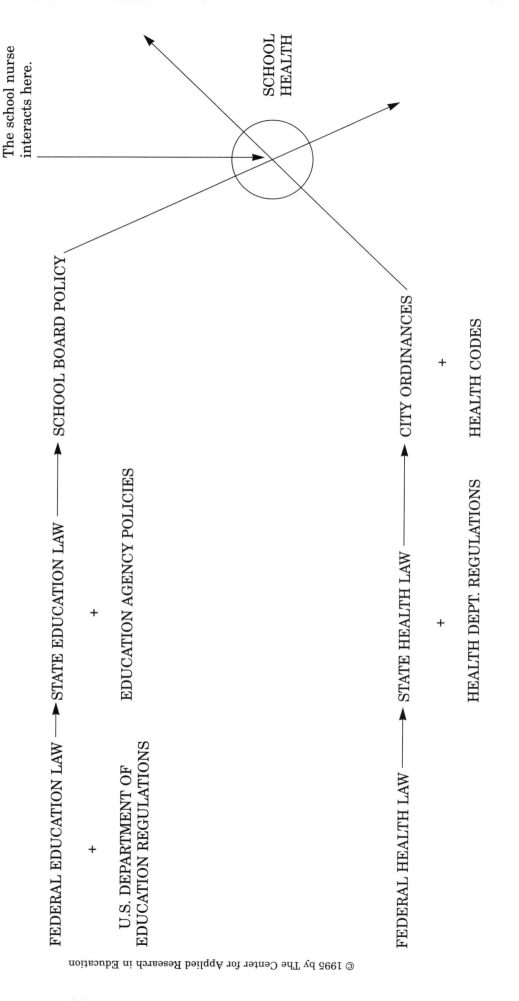

FEDERAL EDUCATION LAW ──▶ STATE EDUCATION LAW ──▶ SCHOOL BOARD POLICY

\+

U.S. DEPARTMENT OF EDUCATION REGULATIONS

\+

EDUCATION AGENCY POLICIES

SCHOOL HEALTH

The school nurse interacts here.

FEDERAL HEALTH LAW ──▶ STATE HEALTH LAW ──▶ CITY ORDINANCES

\+

HEALTH DEPT. REGULATIONS

\+

HEALTH CODES

Figure 12-2

SOURCES OF LEGAL GUIDELINES FOR SCHOOL NURSES

	HEALTH	EDUCATION
FEDERAL/ NATIONAL	Occupational Safety and Health Administration (OSHA)	Individuals with Disabilities Education Act (IDEA)
		Family Education Rights & Privacy Act (FERPA)
	Section 504 of the Rehabilitation Act	Supreme Court Cases
	Americans with Disabilities Act (ADA)	
	ANA Standards	U.S. Department of Education Rules
	NASN Policy Statements	
STATE	Nurse Practice Act	State Education Code
	Medical Practice Act	Court Cases
	Pharmacy Act	
	State Board of Nurse Examiners	Board of Education Policy
	State Nursing Association	Education Agency Regulations
LOCAL	City Health Code/Ordinances	Board of Education Policies
	School Board Policies on Health	
	School Nurse Job Description	
	School Health Department Guidelines and Procedures	School District Administrative Regulations

Figure 12-3a

STUDENT HEALTH RECORD

NOTE: This page of the health record may be copied and forwarded to other school districts without parent permission.

5-14-63
Form H-65—60M—7/06—03-E

NAME: _____ SEX: M___ F___

I.D. # _____ DOB: _____

GRADE/SECTION (Use pencil) _____

FATHER'S NAME: _____

MOTHER'S NAME: _____

ADDRESS: _____ (Work — mother)

PHONE: (Home) _____ (Work — father)

LIVES WITH: _____

HEALTH RECORD

MEDICAL ALERT _____

IMMUNIZATIONS	DATES					
	1st	2nd	3rd	B	B	B
Diphtheria/Tetanus						
Polio						
Measles — Rubeola						
Rubella						
Mumps						
Other						
Verifying Physician						

HEARING

Date						
Hearing R						
Puretone L						
Examiner's Name						
Date						
Ears						
Canals						
T.M.'s						
Immittance Hearing						
Examiner's Name						

VISION

Date of Vision Test					
Vision Test	R 20/	20/	20/	20/	20/
	L 20/	20/	20/	20/	20/
Vision With Glasses	R 20/	20/	20/	20/	20/
	L 20/	20/	20/	20/	20/
COLOR TEST					
PLUS LENS					
HIRSCH-BERG					
Examiner's Name					
Spinal Screening	Date:	Results:		Date:	Results:

Figure 12-3b

NOTE: This page of the health record may NOT be copied or shared without written permission from student's parents.

PHYSICAL EXAMINATION/HEALTH APPRAISAL OR SCREENING

Name _____ D.O.B. _____ I.D.# _____

	PK	K	1	2	3	4	5	6	7	8	9	10	11	12
Grade														
School														
School Year														
Assessment Date														
Medical Code														
Height														
Weight														
*Head Circumference														
Blood Pressure														
General/Skin														
Head/Scalp														
*Eyes/Funduscopy														
*Ears/TMs/Canals														
*Neck														
Nose														
Throat														
Mouth/Teeth														
*Chest/Breasts														
*Lungs														
*Heart/Pulses														
*Abdomen														
Back/Spine														
Extremities/Joints														
*Reflexes														
Balance/Coordination														
*Cranial Nerves														
*Genitalia														
Examiner's Name														

*Included in physical examination

CODE — No Defect Noted   X   Not Correctable   P   Physical Examination
      ✓   Defect Noted   ®   Referred   H   Health Appraisal
      Ø   Corrected   DNT   Did not test

Figure 12-3c

NOTE: This page of the health record may NOT be copied or shared without written permission from student's parents.

Name _____

Birth Date _____

	PROBLEM LIST	Date Inactive/ Resolved	PROGRESS NOTES (2)
Date Entered			Date

PROGRESS NOTES (1)

Date

Figure 12-4

RESOLUTION
HUMAN AND CIVIL RIGHTS FOR STUDENTS

WHEREAS   the capacity to learn may be severely limited by environmental factors or damaged irreversibly by illness or malnutrition; and

WHEREAS   unhealthful environmental conditions and discrimination can generate feelings of rejection and inferiority which can lead to misunderstandings; and

WHEREAS   studies of the at-risk populations of our nation have pointed to the high rate of health problems suffered by these groups;

THEREFORE, BE IT RESOLVED that the National Association of School Nurses believes that all children have the basic human right to a comprehensive school health program to enable them to take full advantage of learning experiences; and

BE IT FURTHER RESOLVED that the National Association of School Nurses strongly recommends that all federally funded school programs for at-risk students include a health component because equal educational opportunity is impossible without attention to health needs.

National Association of School Nurses

Adopted June 1972; Revised June 1982; Revised June 1990

Figure 12-5

RESOLUTION
HUMAN AND CIVIL RIGHTS FOR SCHOOL NURSES

WHEREAS   students can be better prepared to live in a pluralistic world by a staff reflecting the composition of our multi-ethnic society; and

WHEREAS   school nurses have a firm preparation and education in human relations skills;

THEREFORE, BE IT RESOLVED   that the National Association of School Nurses supports active recruitment, employment and retention of minority school nurses with equal promotional opportunities; and

BE IT FURTHER RESOLVED   that the National Association of School Nurses is committed to provide assistance to its members when there are violations of their civil rights or human rights in recruitment, employment, advancement or retention on the educational team.

National Association of School Nurses

Adopted June 1973; Revised June 1982

CHAPTER 13

HIGH-RISK YOUTH

Chapter 13

HIGH-RISK YOUTH

What's done to children, they will do to society.

—*Karl Menninger*

"High-risk" or "at-risk" students, from an educator's perspective, are young people likely to drop out of school or at least engage in behaviors that result in underachievement. From the health professional's point of view, "at-risk" covers a broader spectrum, ranging from death due to reckless or suicidal behaviors, to early unwanted pregnancy and criminal offenses. As the school nurse, you have perhaps, the broadest view of these devastating problems of youth. Your challenge is to find ways to make a difference.

Making a difference means working on at least three levels: (1) helping youngsters one at a time; (2) working with small groups, such as pregnant students; and (3) participating in program planning for large groups of students. It is extremely important that you recognize the common roots of many high-risk behaviors and look for early indicators. This chapter will help you move further in that direction.

PROFILE OF THE 14-YEAR-OLD

To understand some of the whys of teen risk taking we must understand normal adolescent development. I have chosen the 14-year-old to illustrate the beginnings of rapid change toward adult autonomy.

Fourteen is a time of verve and vigor. Boundless energy combines with enthusiasm and goodwill to encourage a boy or girl to attempt almost anything. Friends of both sexes delight. School is okay and extracurricular activities abound. The esteem for parents has faded and the approval of peers is foremost. Yet, the 14-year-old is still very much a part of the family—even though parents frequently embarrass. For the boy especially, it is a time of needing more attention and affection than he can allow himself to accept. Parental efforts to improve behavior are perceived as "bugging." There is a vast difference between the way an ordinary 14-year-old behaves in relation to his or her family and the way he or she relates to the rest of the world. Outside the home, they are unappreciative of family. Boys and girls tend to have a whole crowd of friends; both choose friends partly on the basis of activity interests and partly (especially girls) on the basis of shared interest in the opposite sex. More than half of both sexes are "going steady." Most will say they "make out," and many claim they or their friends have "gone all the way."

Enigmatically, 14-year-olds demonstrate an easy ability to relate to adults, yet see them as relatively unimportant in the scheme of things. They are trying to reconcile their parents' teachings about right and wrong with what their friends do; the result is peer pressure.

Health is good and little school is missed because of illness. At this age, the vast majority say some of their friends drink or use drugs. Alcohol, tobacco, and marijuana are the drugs most frequently reported; amphetamines are also reported. Headaches may occur when demands for adjustment to the environment cannot be met. Reading, in addition to that required for school, is often confined to magazines. Many girls report premenstrual symptoms; most have menstruated by their fourteenth year.

This is the period of most rapid height growth for boys. Deepening of the voice has become more noticeable and the body is more heavily muscled. Lack of self-consciousness may suddenly switch to extreme modesty. By the end of the fourteenth year, most boys experience ejaculation in one situation or another: masturbation is common and nocturnal emissions begin to occur. Fourteen is an age when further sex education is both needed and eagerly received. Styles of dress vary with the region and the latest fad, but within the limits of what everyone else is wearing. Some girls go overboard in their purchase of clothes and use of cosmetics.

Some 14-year-olds spend considerable time in their rooms but most use them only for sleeping and studying. Mood swings are common. Realization dawns that as one gets older life gets more complicated. Sudden flare-ups of temper that seem out of proportion to the occasion occur. Social life (dating; getting something new to wear) gives the greatest happiness. Most 14-year-olds want more freedom and are sure that friends' parents grant it.

Fourteens are willing to face their faults even though they are not good at overcoming them. Money and what money can buy are often wished for; paramount is the desire to have or at least drive a car.

They play around with the thought of the future but say they haven't made up their minds. Fourteens, on the whole, are not eager to marry, recognizing that they have much to do before that time will come. Another realization occurs: Looks are something; intelligence is something, but it's how well two people relate that is of prime importance. Fourteen is thinking realistically about future children; many boys and girls want to have them, but recognize the uncertainties of life.

Girls prefer parties with older boys because they are less rowdy and more mature. Music and video games are an important part of life as are the telephone and television.

Fourteens have the capacity to think in terms of a whole year, relating their interests to the season. Learning through error comes into play more. Though still conformists, aware that they must obey rules, they are now developing their own concepts of morals. Cheating is not usually a problem with well-adjusted fourteens; fairness of teachers is vital.

Concerning school, counselors report several recurring concerns of entering junior high students:

- getting lost; not finding a classroom
- fights; being teased
- vandalism of personal property
- others getting them in trouble
- being put in suspension
- pressure to be cool
- getting to know kids from other schools
- getting yelled at in public
- not being popular
- which teachers are nice
- getting long and boring assignments
- getting bad grades
- bad lunches

Most of the items on this list reflect the commonality of wanting to do well in school, but it is evident there are many developmental tasks to perform, with distractions along the way.

TEEN PARENTHOOD

Overview

Several sources agree that approximately one million adolescent pregnancies occur in this country annually. Half of these result in live births while the other half end in miscarriages or abortions. Teen pregnancy is, by any definition, an epidemic.

Once a young person experiences coitus, she or he acquires "risk status." Unquestionably, young people who are not sexually active are not at risk of pregnancy, unless they are forced to have sex (not a rare event). Once the decision is made to initiate sexual activity, risk of pregnancy is high for those who do not use contraception consistently. Once pregnant, a young woman must decide whether to carry the pregnancy to term. She may decide on an abortion, if that option is available to her. If a child is born, the mother may decide to give the child up for adoption.

While this series of decisions seems relatively straightforward, there is little consensus in our society about how to intervene and prevent the negative consequences. One set of conflicts centers on the morality of premarital sex. Some people believe that the only response to the issue of adolescent pregnancy is to promote abstention. Others believe that premarital sexual activity has become the norm and, therefore, interventions should focus on teaching responsible sexual behavior and providing access to contraception. A second set of conflicts is focused on the abortion issue. Once pregnant, should a girl be required to maintain the pregnancy and encouraged to put the baby up for adoption if she cannot care for it, or should she be assisted to obtain an abortion if that is what she wants?

Role of Young Males

Our knowledge of the role of young males in sexuality and pregnancy behaviors is incomplete. Much of the published information on adolescent pregnancy ignores males, except to acknowledge that they are "perpetrators" of the outcomes.

Information about almost 40% of the fathers of babies born to teenage mothers is missing from vital statistics. Close to 70% of the identified fathers are over the age of 19. No data are available about the age of the male partners in teen pregnancies that terminate in abortions, but it is probable that those males are younger than the fathers of live births. In any case, males must be included in target populations for pregnancy prevention programs.

Consequences of Early Pregnancy

Early sexual intercourse places young women at very high risk of negative health consequences. The younger the age at which a girl first enters into sexual relationships, the more likely that negative consequences will follow. Early sexual initiates have more frequent acts of coitus and multiple partners, and are less likely to use effective methods of contraception. The most deleterious consequences, other than pregnancy, are sexually transmitted diseases and their related side effects (infertility, cervical cancer, ectopic pregnancy, and infections passed on to newborns). AIDS is the most life-threatening consequence; young people who are involved in an array of high-risk behaviors, such as drug use, prostitution, and frequent sex with multiple partners, are extremely vulnerable.

The most direct consequences of early pregnancy relate to childbearing. The birth of a child impacts both the mother and the baby—and ultimately the father, family, and community—with immediate, long-term, and often lifetime, consequences. Very young mothers, under the age of 15, suffer the worst physical effects, with heightened risks of complications and mortality. Teen mothers under the age of 18 are more likely to have toxemia, anemia, and prolonged labor. Their babies are at higher risk of prematurity and low birthweight that in turn often produce developmental delays.

In the years following early childbearing, teen mothers suffer several disadvantages: reduced educational achievement, unstable marriages and high divorce rates, or no marriage, more subsequent births closer together and unintended, lower-status jobs, lower incomes and, in some cases, long-term welfare dependency. Adverse effects on children of teen parents include lower achievement, many more behavioral and emotional problems, high risk of becoming teenage parents themselves, and often, a lifetime of poverty.

Adoption is a decision that teens rarely make following unplanned pregnancies. No studies have been identified that document the psychological consequences of adoption, such as depression or regret, although it undoubtedly occurs in some cases. There is no evidence in the psychological literature that abortion produces depression or guilt. Most anecdotal reports refer to feelings of relief.

Precursors of High-Risk Behavior

The target behaviors considered high risk are (1) early sexual activity, (2) nonuse, or inconsistent use of contraceptives, and (3) early childbearing. Many of the precursors are the same for each of these three high-risk behaviors. Figure 13-1, located at the end of this chapter, is a tabulation of the precursors of early childbearing.

African-American young people, especially boys, are more likely to have intercourse at very early ages. Early pubertal development has some influence on age of initiation. Young people from low-income families with uneducated parents who are not supportive or communicative are much more likely to initiate sex at early ages. Children who are not engaged in school activities, who have low expectations for school achievement, and who hang around with friends in similar situations are more prone to early sex. This behavior is often preceded by other high-risk behaviors, such as early substance use and truancy. They are often drawn into gangs, prostitution, and the underground economy of stolen goods and drug trafficking.

The living room couch has long since displaced the back seat of the car or the beach as the place of intercourse. The use of contraception follows a pattern that is linked to early initiation of intercourse and other behaviors. Hispanics are less likely to use contraception either initially or subsequently. Young, sexually active teens who do not use contraception are more impulsive and lack an internalized locus of control; they are poor planners. They are more likely to have casual sex and not be in committed relationships with partners. Their parents have limited education and are less likely to communicate with them or may have been early parents themselves.

Girls who bear children early appear to have limited basic life skills; pregnancy just seems to happen to them. Some are less cognitively able than their peers; some are submissive and depressed. Others use marriage or pregnancy as a way to escape an unsupportive family and create someone who will love them. And, most sadly, many early pregnancies are the result of sexual abuse.

Prevention of Adolescent Pregnancy

Family Interventions

There is no substitute for a supportive, involved family when it comes to primary prevention of teen pregnancy. Strong evidence supports the theory that good parent-child communication helps children improve their decision making skills and delays intercourse. Schools can give suggestions for parent involvement with their children and reinforce good parenting; your input is vital in this area.

School-Based Interventions

The school's role in minimizing the negative impact of teen pregnancy comes under three headings: curriculum, counseling, and school-based clinics.

That sex education improves knowledge has been well documented, but there is little evidence that behavior is influenced by taking courses. The rate of sexual activity does not appear to change as a result of information, nor does contraceptive use. There is no evidence that pregnancies have been prevented as an outcome of any specific sex education curriculum. Sex educators have responded to these disappointing research results by developing new approaches, such as decision-making skills and life planning. The jury is still out, but this approach holds more promise.

The term, *Counseling,* encompasses a wide variety of activities, from advice for an impacted individual to generic, "preventive" sessions for groups. The essential element for success seems to be a one-on-one relationship between the student and an adult. Such a relationship must be ongoing so that rapport and trust can be developed. The "one-minute psychologist" approach does not work; written handouts and a pat on the back are valueless, unless followed up. The adult must truly care what happens to the child—and show it frequently.

School-Based Clinics

The number of school-based and school-linked health clinics is increasing— as is their acceptance. A broad view will be presented in Chapter 14, but in the context of sexually active adolescents, these clinics have the most documentable track record of reducing teen pregnancy—especially second and third pregnancies. The success of school-based clinics seems to hinge on the fact that they are comprehensive health centers and see adolescents for any number of problems— not just family planning. They reach a higher percentage of youth in a given population, especially males. Most school-based clinics report that student visits related to family planning constitute only about 15 percent of visits. No stigma accompanies a school clinic visit; peers need not know the reason. A student's confidential problems are often unknown to school personnel unless there is a need to know—such as schedule adjustment. School nurses sometimes resent this, but sharing of information between the school and an on-campus clinic run by another agency must be worked out at the local level.

As the school nurse, you can and should perform a supportive role in monitoring pregnant students. See Figure 13-2. Because of the high incidence of complications in expectant mothers under the age of 16, your checks between prenatal visits can assist with early intervention. Figure 13-3 is an example of a health care monitoring and counseling record for pregnant students. All pertinent information can be recorded in four pages.

Contraception

Because condoms are often forgotten or not used in the "heat of the moment," and daily pills are difficult to remember and have side effects, more health care professionals are prescribing long-acting contraceptives such as Norplant and Depo-Provera injections.

Emergency contraception (EC)—also known as post-coital contraception or the "morning after" pill—was first used in Europe for rape victims. One type of EC, the Yuzpe method, involves taking four estrogen/progestin pills: two tablets taken at 12-hour intervals within 72 hours of unprotected intercourse. British women will soon be able to buy these combination pills over the counter. Although it is not available in America yet, RU-486, an estrogen/progestin preparation, is being studied by one pharmaceutical company. The faculty at Northwestern Medical School (Chicago) estimates that this method could reduce the number of unintended pregnancies by 1.76 million and the number of abortions by 0.8 million.

VIOLENCE

Scope of the Problem

Statistics abound to document increasing violence in this country. Once limited to urban areas, it is now infesting suburban and rural communities. Numerous student homicides make it impossible to minimize the impact of violence on the schools. In New York City, homicide is now the number-one cause of death among young males. The 26th Annual Phi Delta Kappa/Gallup Poll of Public

Attitudes Toward Public Schools (1994) for the first time placed violence and lack of discipline as the top two concerns. Figure 13-4 gives the causes of death for males ages 15–34.

The School's Role

The causes of violence are multifactoral, complex, and not entirely understood. Of those causes thought to be understood, few are controlled by schools, yet schools must take steps to prevent and control all types of violence. Foremost must be the physical safety of students and staff while on campus. If students don't live, nothing else matters.

Broad areas of intervention that can be undertaken by schools include

- safe school environment (e.g., identification badges and metal detectors)
- staff modeling of civil behavior (e.g., abolishing corporal punishment)
- peer mediation (let students attempt to resolve their own conflicts)
- violence prevention curricula (e.g., Prothrow-Stith; see references)
- drug education
- gang prevention and control (e.g., cooperation with police gang units)

As with other high-risk behaviors, the foundation is laid in early childhood. The opening epigram of this chapter says a lot: "What's done to children, they will do to society." If all family conflicts result in physical blows between members, the child's repertoire of skills for de-escalating violence is severely limited. The first step schools must take in the prevention of violence is to stop corporal punishment if it still has this policy, because it sends the wrong message to students. Figure 13-5 is NASN's resolution on corporal punishment. Beyond physical security measures and staff modeling, the schools' best hope for breaking the violence cycle probably lies in peer mediation programs and early violence prevention curricula.

Peer Mediation

Peer mediation most commonly involves arbitration between two conflicted students by a third, disinterested student who is specially trained and often a year older. Impressive results have been obtained by placing a troublesome student in the role of arbiter. Tremendous insight is gained by the arbiter when he or she brings a dispute to a win-win conclusion.

Violence Prevention Curricula

Currently, the most-used violence prevention curriculum is Debra Prothrow-Stith's *Violence Prevention Curriculum for Adolescents* (see references). Although designed for high school students, it is being used by many schools at the junior high level. The basic lessons are

- There is a lot of violence in society.
- Anger is normal.
- There are healthy ways to express anger.
- There is more to lose than gain from fighting.
- Saving face is important.

Communitywide Efforts

Violence prevention efforts must intervene at every possible point—in all facets of society and at various developmental stages for the individual child. The earliest intervention begins with parenting skills. Parents should create a calm and just environment and avoid corporal punishment, but set reasonable limits. Short of physical abuse, inconsistent application of rules is the most devastating; it's impossible to believe in the rules if they are always changing. Consistency is the watchword for all ages. Many community agencies offer parenting programs. Parenting classes for teenage mothers can also be the school's starting point.

All the studies on children and television violence conducted over the last 30 years point to the same finding: television violence is directly linked to children's using violence themselves. The impact of television violence can be controlled at two points: programming and viewing. The major networks are now looking carefully at the violence content of children's programs. Unquestionably, parents should control the viewing of their children; Saturday morning cartoons are far from violence free.

Police gang units are beginning to show successful results in their role as information clearing house and rumor control center. Gangs are beginning to trust them as reliable sources of information and the rates of retaliation homicides are dropping as a result of their efforts.

Gun control is on the national agenda and making headway despite the NRA. Research clearly shows that the availability of guns strongly influences the number of homicides and that drugs and alcohol are strongly linked to both homicides and motor vehicle deaths.

Primary and Secondary Prevention

Primary prevention of violence is the goal, but it cannot be attained without strong families. Again, parenting skills are the most crucial element. In secondary prevention, the schools are the key agency because they are involved with all children and adolescents. Schools must embrace this role with vigor, for without a calm, supportive learning environment, other educational efforts count for naught.

The last-ditch violence control measure is incarceration—a sometimes necessary tertiary prevention effort. Penal rehabilitation efforts are not generally successful, although there is a handful of positive outcomes.

SUBSTANCE ABUSE

The Current Scene

Research findings on the etiology of substance abuse are beginning to reveal some clear findings regarding the antecedents and consequences of substance abuse; yet it is still difficult to sort out "non-risk" experimentation. Only certain subsets of students who currently use substances get into any trouble as a result of their experimentation; that is, the concept of gateway drugs (tobacco and alcohol) has limited usefulness in identifying adolescents who will become serious users. Not every young person needs to be in the target population for intensive prevention efforts. We must look for the subsets at greatest risk and invest our time and money there. These subsets are sizable as reflected in the estimates of Dryfoos (reference #3) for 10 to 17-year-olds:

- use tobacco product   17%
- drink alcohol fairly often   32%
- use marijuana   11%
- tried cocaine   3%

These estimates are not additive, since much of substance abuse involves multiple substances. Of these youth at risk, many are already established smokers and heavy drinkers. The crack form of cocaine, which is smoked, is the most quickly addicting substance yet identified; some experts say it takes only one experience.

There is a growing consensus among researchers about the precursors of substance-abusing behavior: early initiation and susceptibility to peer influence are significant markers. Interestingly, the other end of the conformity spectrum, extreme nonconformity, also predisposes young people to substance abuse. Other significant patterns include rebelliousness and independence, school underachievement, and absenteeism. Eventually these translate into low aspirations for further education and may culminate in dropping out of school.

Protective Factors

Family, peers, school, and community all play a role in protecting young people against drug abuse. Key protective factors in each of these areas include:

- Family
  - Seeks prenatal care
  - Manages stress well
  - Uses high warmth/low criticism parenting
  - Values and encourages education

- –Has clear expectations
- –Encourages supportive relationship with caring adults beyond the family
- –Shares family responsibilities
- Peers
  - –Involved in drug-free activities
  - –Respect authority
  - –Bonded to conventional groups
  - –Appreciate the unique talents of individuals
- School
  - –Has high expectations
  - –Views itself as nurturing
  - –Fosters active involvement of students
  - –Involves parents
  - –Trains teachers in social development
  - –Provides drug-free alternative activities
- Community
  - –Policies and norms support nonuse among youth
  - –Provides access to resources (housing, health care, child care, recreation, job training, and employment)
  - –Involves youth in community service
  - –Provides supportive networks and social bonds

The African proverb, "it takes a whole village to raise a child," clearly applies to American communities trying to prevent high-risk behaviors of all kinds. The support and intervention network must permeate all aspects of a child's life from birth on.

Intervention Programs

An analysis of 143 adolescent drug prevention programs by Tobler (1986) confirmed some of our early suspicions. Three-fourths of the programs were in junior high schools and one-fourth at the high school level. The interventions fell into one or more of five categories of prevention strategies:

- knowledge oriented only
- affective strategies only
- social influence and life skills (peer influence)
  - –refusal skills
  - –social and life skills

- knowledge plus affective strategies
- alternative strategies
  - –introduce activities
  - –teach competence in high risk youth

The programs in aggregate had the most effect on knowledge—twice that of any other variable, but they had relatively little effect on changing attitudes. Tobler found the effect on changes in substance use was only half the size of the effect on knowledge changes. This change in use was much greater for cigarette smoking than other substances. Of the five models studied, social influence and life skills (peer influence programs) had the greatest effect on all outcome measures. The alternative programs were second most effective, but the effect was only half that of the social influence programs. Does this mean we should give up the drug education curriculum in the classroom? Probably not, since accurate information is needed to make informed decisions. It means we need more than knowledge to change behavior.

When the best preventive efforts fail, we need the safety net of drug treatment programs. As pointed out in Chapter 4, schools can promote the treatment of drug abusing students by making referrals to specialized centers and by not invoking punitive measures against first offenders who agree to treatment.

CHILD ABUSE AND NEGLECT

Definition, Prevalence, and Symptoms

Great strides have been made in recognizing and intervening in cases of child abuse since the enactment of the Child Abuse Prevention and Treatment Act of 1974. The act defined child abuse as

> . . . physical or mental injury, sexual abuse, negligent treatment, or maltreatment of a child under the age of 18 by a person who is responsible for the child's welfare under circumstances which indicate the child's health or welfare is harmed or threatened thereby.

In addition to defining abuse, the legislation established the national Center on Child Abuse and required that persons who *suspected* abusive practices report them to Child Protective Services. Proof was not required—merely suspicion.

Statistics documenting levels of abuse are difficult to obtain and verify for accuracy because of unevenness in reporting practices. It is estimated that 1.5 million children, between the ages of 3 and 17 are the victims of violent behavior each year. Figures from child protective services are lower, probably due to underreporting.

School personnel, especially teachers and school nurses, who spend 30 hours a week with children, are the most frequent reporters of child abuse.

The most common symptom of physical abuse is bruising—especially multiple bruises in various stages of healing and bruises in unusual places. Other findings suggestive of abuse are welts, cuts, or punctures of the skin; hot liquid burns; and cigarette burns.

Abusive Parents

Sexual abuse is more difficult to suspect as schools do not routinely examine the genitalia. Child behaviors that suggest the possibility of sexual abuse include

- unusually aggressive or withdrawn behavior
- unusual apprehension with adults
- frequent severe mood changes
- premature sexual behavior, such as rubbing against adults

School personnel should also be aware of personality characteristics of fathers who sexually abuse their daughters:

- introverted personality with minimal extrafamilial social contact
- inability to form close attachments with spouse and children
- general immaturity

Wives in incestuous families may either exhibit immaturity and passive dependency or actively encourage the incestuous relationship to cover up their own promiscuity.

Physically abusive parents of both sexes often display excessively punitive disciplinary practices, even in public, and rarely show affection toward their children. Other parents, especially those who have been reported in the past for suspected abuse, may make a show of affection in public.

Long-Term Effects

Review of matched studies of abused and nonabused children reveal that the abused children suffer social, emotional, and intellectual difficulties. The abused child is more likely to have a learning disorder.

Results of self-image questionnaires administered to female adolescent sexual abuse victims showed many more indicators of psychiatric problems than matched controls: emotional liability, poor impulse control, and few coping skills. A history of early sexual abuse is common among prostitutes.

Several studies conclude that victims of child abuse are more likely to exhibit violent behavior and become abusive parents themselves. Child neglect, while more subtle and often less severe, can also have disastrous results—particularly if a child has an underlying medical condition such as diabetes or asthma.

We are just beginning to understand the long term effects of child abuse and neglect. Many more psychological studies are needed to provide a complete and accurate picture.

Prevention and Intervention

Attempts at primary prevention of child abuse frustrate professionals because not all families can be monitored. We know that abusive injuries resulting in death are usually preceded by one or more previous reports of abuse. Thus, vigorous secondary prevention is extremely productive if child protective services are funded at a level that allows investigation of all reports.

School personnel must make their assessment of risk known to child protective services. If a situation is felt to be life threatening, or to involve sexual abuse, it must be so stated in writing. School nurses should follow up with an inquiry when their reports are not investigated. Reporting fulfills your legal obligation, but does not complete your moral and ethical obligation as a child advocate.

Nurses can also push for parenting skills courses for all students, but particularly for teenage parents in their school systems. Such courses probably hold the most promise for impacting primary prevention in the school setting.

HIV AND HEPATITIS B

Professionals and laypeople alike now realize that HIV infection progresses to full-blown AIDS and ultimately death, although the time sequence is variable. In contrast, most of the laity and certainly the majority of adolescents do not realize that hepatitis B is transmitted in a manner identical to that for HIV, that is, sexually and by contact with blood. Nor do they realize that chronic progressive or recurrent liver disease is common with hepatitis B and may lead to cirrhosis and death.

As with teen pregnancy, the only effective primary prevention lies in sexual abstinence. Short of this, condoms are highly effective in reducing both pregnancy and sexually transmitted diseases (STD). Misconceptions regarding birth control pills abound among teenagers. Many females and males falsely believe that contraceptive pills prevent STD. Some teens are learning the truth the hard way when they contract gonorrhea, but it is a valuable lesson if it impacts future sexual behavior.

The adolescent mind-set of immortality is difficult to combat. Even if they understand the facts of transmission, they are likely to say to themselves, "It won't happen to me," or "Even if it does, I'll be the one to beat it." This may be one area, along with drunk driving, where so-called scare tactics are indicated, particularly since nothing else seems to work when adequate family support is lacking.

COMMON ROOTS OF HIGH-RISK BEHAVIORS

Teen parenthood, STD, substance abuse, delinquency, and violence share six common characteristics that predict each of the problem behaviors (Dryfoos 1990).

Age: Early initiation of risk behavior predicts more negative consequences.

Education: All problem behaviors are associated with doing poorly in school.

Behavior: Acting out, truancy, antisocial behavior, and conduct disorders are related to each of the problem behaviors.

Peers: Having low resistance to peer influences and having friends who participate in the same behaviors are common to all of the behaviors.

Parents: Having parents who do not monitor, offer guidance, or communicate with their children, and having parents who are either too authoritarian or too permissive are all strongly associated with the behaviors.

Neighborhood: Living in a poverty area, or an urban, high-density community is predictive of these problems.

Much has been said of households headed by single females, but the research suggests that it is more the quality of the parenting than the composition of the family. One nurturing parent or caretaker can be a more significant influence than two nonnurturing parents.

Depression and related stress are documented precursors of school dropout and substance abuse. Another common factor underlying all these behaviors is nonconformity—as measured by lower religiosity, tolerance of deviance, more liberal views, peer approval of deviant behavior, and poor school performance.

If one creates a composite from national surveys it reveals the following risk groups for 11- to 17-year-olds:

Very high risk (heavy drug use; delinquency)	=	11%
Moderate risk (alcohol or marijuana; sexually active; minor offenses)	=	40%
Low/no risk (not sexually active; rarely or never use drugs)	=	49%

The most consistent precursor to all these problem behaviors is school underachievement, which frequently leads to dropping out. This is borne out by data from the juvenile justice system, which shows that 85% of juvenile offenders who appear in court are illiterate.

The strong positive association between substance use of any kind and early sexual activity has been well documented. As an example, marijuana users are nine times more likely to be sexually active than nonusers.

The reasons dropouts give for leaving school provide further support for the commonality of underachievement: 82% of the girls and 100% of the boys cite a school-related reason, such as poor grades or dislike of school. While the conventional wisdom has been that girls drop out of school because of pregnancy, recent analyses suggest that many girls who become mothers drop out prior to the pregnancy.

No one study has analyzed precisely how the various separate behaviors are interrelated, but the overlap is obvious.

- Early initiation of smoking and alcohol leads to heavier use of cigarettes and alcohol, and also leads to the use of marijuana and other illicit drugs.
- Heavy substance abuse is associated with early sexual activity, lower grades, dropping out, and delinquency.
- Delinquency is associated with early sexual activity, early pregnancy, substance abuse, low grades, and dropping out.
- Early initiation of sexual activity is related to the use of cigarettes and alcohol, use of marijuana and other illicit drugs, lower grades, dropping out, and delinquency.
- Early childbearing is related to early sexual activity, heavy drug use, low academic achievement, dropping out, and delinquency.
- School failure leads to dropping out. Lower grades are associated with substance use and early childbearing. Truancy and school misbehavior are related to substance abuse, dropping out, and delinquency.
- Drugs and alcohol are strongly linked to homicides and motor vehicle deaths.

Again, *school failure seems to be the initial event*. Once that occurs, other events begin to take place. Doing poorly in school and minor delinquent offenses seem to fit together, and as high-risk children grow older, substance abuse and sexual activity enter the picture along with their negative consequences.

To summarize, young people who exhibit two or more high-risk behaviors often share many of these characteristics:

- doing poorly in school
- starting any of the behaviors early
- acting out
- associating with friends who act out
- having inattentive parents
- living in a disadvantaged neighborhood

Minority status and low socioeconomic status (SES) compound these behaviors in some, but not all, cases.

The message seems clear: Move away from the traditional categorical approaches to intervention and begin to design a more comprehensive approach. The identification of common predictors of multiple-problem behaviors lends force to the argument that interventions should focus more on the *predictors* of the behavior than on the behavior itself. Another consideration in prevention programs is the extent to which predictors are *amenable to intervention;* if you can't influence them, why waste time and money? If there is a developmental progression, it is also necessary to identify *key* events for early intervention. These requirements lead to the conclusion that enhancement of early schooling and prevention of school failure should receive high priority not only from those interested in lowering the dropout rate but also from those interested in preventing substance abuse, pregnancy, violence, and delinquency.

The new focus of grants from the federal level calls for programs to achieve multiple rather than single goals (i.e., dropout prevention, pregnancy prevention, and drug abuse prevention). Prevention strategy must be centered in schools because that's where the children are and because school failure is the first domino to fall in the cascade of high-risk behaviors. Community agencies should be allowed to bring their services into schools and work in tandem with student support services.

The business world now perceives the wisdom of contributing to the effort to stop the downward spiral of academic performance, for they will inherit the inferior product and pay for it later.

A clinical study of formerly incarcerated male delinquents (average age = 16) by Dorothy Othow Lewis (1994) tells the sad second chapter for many school dropouts:

> Follow-up clinical interviews were administered to subjects, approximately 9 years after discharge from juvenile corrections. All but six of 97 had adult criminal records, most for violent crimes. Only 10% were graduated from high school; 30% received minimal job training; most worked sporadically at unskilled jobs. Few married. Although 35 had fathered children, only five were living with them. Psychiatric treatment for identified vulnerabilities was negligible. Upon discharge, the most neuropsychiatrically impaired and violent subjects tended to be placed in adult corrections; the most intact were placed in special schools and psychiatric hospitals. Placement in families was associated with fewer adult aggressive offenses than was institutional placement. Based on their well-documented early vulnerabilities and needs, this sample of delinquents did not obtain the kinds of supports subsequent to juvenile incarceration that might have enabled them to function independently in society.

YOUR CONTRIBUTION

We are back again to considering the whole child. Most categorical programs (e.g., drug abuse education, pregnancy prevention) have been only marginally successful, with too little too late. As school nurse you are one of the few people who potentially interact with every student in the school. You are often the first one turned to in cases of teen pregnancy and drug abuse. You can use your influence to urge schools to develop *comprehensive,* rather than categorical, programs to deal with the *antecedents* of high-risk behaviors collectively rather than wait until the behaviors appear, to be dealt with by separate programs. One student with three high-risk behaviors should not have to seek help from three different service units.

In addition to being comprehensive, high-risk prevention programs should begin at the early elementary level, involve peers and parents, and be flexible. You can be a spokesperson for lowering the fences of turfism and giving more than lip service to the multidisciplinary approach.

SUMMARY

We have looked at a number of pigeonholed issues and tried to recognize some etiologic commonalities. Certainly, school personnel influence only a small number of variables in a child's life. Much of personality has been molded by parents and others at home before a child enters school. Nevertheless, the school's impact is not small. There are enough success stories to keep us searching for the one moment for each youth when the door opens and lets in the future.

REFERENCES

1. Cady, J. "Adolescent Males: The Forgotten Half." In *Clinical Issues in Perinatal and Women's Health Nursing: Adolescence.* Philadelphia: J. B. Lippincott, 1991.

2. Dawes, R. *House of Cards: Psychology and Psychotherapy Built on Myth.* New York: The Free Press (Macmillan), 1994.

3. Dryfoos, J. *Adolescents at Risk: Prevalence and Prevention.* New York: Oxford University Press, 1990.

4. Elster, A. *AMA Guidelines for Adolescent Preventive Services (GAPS).* Chicago: American Medical Association, 1994.

5. Hudson, D. "Human Nature, Gender and Ethnicity." In *The Great Ideas Today.* Chicago: Encyclopedia Britannica, 1994.

6. Kohn, R. "The Mystery of the Mind." In *The Great Ideas Today.* Chicago: Encyclopedia Britannica, 1994.

7. Lewis, D. "A Clinical Follow-up of Delinquent Males: Ignored Vulnerabilities, Unmet Needs, and the Perpetuation of Violence." *Journal of the American Academy of Child Adolescent Psychology* 33(4):518, 1994.

8. Orr, D. "Premature Sexual Activity as an Indicator of Psychosocial Risk." *Pediatrics* 87:141–147, 1991.

9. Prothrow-Stith, D. *Violence Prevention Curriculum for Adolescents.* Newton, MA: Education Development Center, 1987.

10. Reece, R. *Child Abuse: Medical Diagnosis and Management.* Philadelphia: Lea and Febiger, 1994.

11. Roth, B. "The School Nurse as Adolescent Health Educator." *Journal of School Nursing,* (Supplement), December 1993.

12. Saylor, C. *Children and Disasters.* New York: Plenum Press, 1993.

13. Spivak, H. "The Role of the Pediatrician in Violence Prevention." *Pediatrics* (Supplement). 94(4):577–649, 1994.

14. Stanton, B. "Adolescent Drug Trafficking." *Pediatrics* (Supplement). 93(6):1039–1084, 1994.

15. ———. "Sexual Practices and Intentions Among Preadolescent and Early Adolescent Low-Income Urban African-Americans." *Pediatrics* 93(6):966–973, 1994.

16. Tobler, N. "Meta-Analysis of 143 Adolescent Drug Prevention Programs." *Journal of Drug Issues* 16: 537–567, 1986.

17. Tyrer, P. *Models for Mental Disorder: Conceptual Models in Psychiatry.* New York: John Wiley and Sons, 1993.

18. U.S. Department of Health and Human Services. *School Health: Findings from Evaluated Programs.* Washington, DC, 1993.

19. Wilde, J. "When Sexual Abuse Is Suspected." *Contemporary Pediatrics* 11:93–102, 1994.

20. Wuthnow, R. *Sharing the Journey: Support Groups and America's New Quest for Community.* New York: The Free Press (Macmillan), 1994.

Figure 13-1

PRECURSORS OF EARLY CHILDBEARING*

Precursor	Early Coitus	Contraceptive nonuse
Educational expectations	low	low
Perception of life options	poor	poor
School grades	low	low
Conduct	truancy	—
Religiosity	low attendance	variable
Peer influence	heavy	—
Peer use	—	imitative
Beliefs about risk	—	unconcerned
Other high-risk behaviors	early delinquency; substance use	—
Psychological factors	—	impulsive
Self-esteem	variable	lack locus of control
Relationship to partner	—	uncommitted

*After Dryfoos.

Figure 13-2

RESOLUTION
SCHOOL-AGE PARENTS

WHEREAS   increasing numbers of adolescents are sexually active and at risk of becoming parents; and

WHEREAS   a high percentage of those females who choose to carry their pregnancy to term are keeping their infants; and

WHEREAS   pregnancy and child rearing responsibilities are the greatest single cause of female high school students' dropping out of school before graduation;

THEREFORE, BE IT RESOLVED that the National Association of School Nurses believes that education should include human reproduction and family planning information in an effort to prepare students to clarify values and make responsible decisions; and

BE IT ALSO RESOLVED that the National Association of School Nurses believes that the school nurse should provide counseling and information regarding pregnancy to young people and their families; and

BE IT FURTHER RESOLVED that the National Associaton of School Nurses believes that the school nurse should support the establishment of child care services and the inclusion of growth and development and parenting education in the school based academic program.

National Association of School Nurses

Adopted 1971; Revised June 1982

Figure 13-3a

HEALTH CARE MONITORING AND COUNSELING RECORD
FOR PREGNANT STUDENTS

Demographic Data:

Name _____ Date _____ Home School _____

Married _____ Husband's Name _____

Address _____ Home Phone _____

Mother's Name _____ Work Phone _____

Address _____

Father's Name _____ Work Phone _____

Address _____

Age _____ D.O.B. _____ LMP _____ EDC _____ Week or Month of Pregnancy _____

Clinic or Physician _____ Phone _____ First Appointment _____

Routine prenatal health care visits are scheduled:　Every four (4) weeks up to 32 weeks (end of this period _____)

write in pencil

Every two (2) weeks up to 36 weeks (end of this period _____)

write in pencil

Then every week until delivery. Record dates for future medical prenatal care. When the appointment has been kept or changed, record the new date. Student to be seen by school nurse approximately midway between Physician/Clinic visits.

Medical Prenatal Appointments

1. ____　2. ____　3. ____　4. ____　5. ____

6. ____　7. ____　8. ____　9. ____　10. ____

11. ____　12. ____　13. ____　14. ____　15. ____

School Prenatal Appointments

1. ____　2. ____　3. ____　4. ____　5. ____

6. ____　7. ____　8. ____　9. ____　10. ____

11. ____　12. ____　13. ____　14. ____　15. ____

HISTORY

I. **Health Problem(s),** during past 12 months: (list and describe management/treatment) Are there other known health problems?

II. **Past History:** (list with date and age)

    A. Hospitalizations — (Include reason) overnight stay, emergency room visit, outpatient, day surgery

    B. Illness — (Including contagious diseases, high fever, etc.)

    C. Injuries — accidents, ingestions, head injury, sequale

    D. Medications —

    E. Allergies —

    F. Last Health Care Visit _____ Name of Provider _____

    Purpose of visit (acute care) (Routine P.E.) _____

    Dental Care　Date of last visit _____ Purpose _____ Provider _____

Figure 13-3b

III. **Family History:**

Biological Father — Age: _____ Health _____

Maternal Grandparents: Paternal Grandparents:

1. Grandmother — Age: _____ Health _____   1. Grandmother Age: _____ Health _____

2. Grandfather — Age: _____ Health _____   2. Grandfather Age: _____ Health _____

Familial Diseases: (circle) Heart Disease, stroke, hypertension, diabetes, asthma, allergy, anemia, sickle cell disease or trait, arthritis, cancer, epilepsy, cataracts, glaucoma, kidney disease, tuberculosis, mental problems, mental retardation, learning problems, other.

(Explain) _____

IV. **Social History:**

Household members:

Housing:

Plans for future:

Child: Adoption   Self: Education
           Keep Child   Parenting Classes
           Child Care Plans   Prenatal Classes
                                                       High School
                                                       Trade School
                                                       College
                                                       Marriage

V. **Post Delivery History:**

Labor and Delivery: Place _____
Length of Labor —
Type of Delivery —
Condition of Mother —
Problems: (circle) breathing, forceps, C-section, other_____
Birth weight _____
Neonatal:
Problems: (circle) breathing, infections, RH factor, jaundice, transfusions, bleeding, congenital anomaly, feeding, other.
(Explain)

Post natal:
Home from the Hospital — Baby in _____ days. Mother in _____ days. Complications —
(Explain)

Return to school _____ Post Partum Check Up _____

Child care arrangements _____ Lives with _____

Figure 13-3c

VI. **Past OB History** (if applicable):

Gravida _____ Para _____ AB _____
(# of Pregnancies)   (# of Live Babies)

_____ Delivery: Vaginal _____ C-Section _____
Date

If C-Section, state reason: _____

Prenatal: Maternal age _____ Length of pregnancy _____ # of pregnancies _____

# of living children _____ #of miscarriages _____ Prenatal care — (where and what month

begun) _____ Habits: (circle) smoking, drinking, drugs, pica, other _____

(Explain) _____

_____

High Risks: (circle) Infections, bleeding, high blood pressure, anemia, fever, RH factor, trauma, inherited

disease(s), medications, weight gain, chronic disease, hospitalization, other: _____

_____

_____

VII. **Review of Systems** (circle)

1. General — Changes in weight, appetite, activity level, bowel habits, resistance to disease, other. (Explain) Birth defects — congenital anomalies

2. Skin — Rashes, easy bruising, changes in skin color or texture, eczema, impetigo, growths, or tumors. (Explain)

3. Head — Headache, trauma, infections (Explain)

4. Eyes — Vision changes, trauma, infections, cataracts, glaucoma, other (Explain)

5. Ears, Nose, Throat — Infections (specify), trauma, epistaxis, allergies, hearing changes, voice changes, canes, speech problems. (Explain)

6. Neck — Trauma, swollen lymph nodes, limitation of movement. (Explain)

7. Respiratory — Infections, breathing problems, trauma, wheezing, cough, asthma (Explain)

8. Cardiovascular — murmur, fatigue with exertion, cyanosis (Explain)

9. Gastrointestinal — Abdominal pain, nausea, jaundice, vomiting, diarrhea, constipation, ulcer. (Explain)

10. Genitourinary — Infections, enuresis, encopresis, discharge, rashes, menstruation, sexual development (Explain)

11. Musculosketal — Trauma, limitation of movement, joint pain or swelling, growths of tumor, curvature of the spine, braces, corrective shoes (explain)

12. Neurological — Birth injury, trauma, seizures (febrile vs. afebrile), staring spells, poor coordination or balance, dizziness, syncope, developmental evaluation (Explain)

13. Endocrine — Increased thirst, appetite, urination, diabetes, thyroid problems (Explain)

14. Hematologic — Anemia, blood transfusions, blood dyscrasias, sickle cell (Explain)

15. Psychosocial — Changes in activity level, behavior, relationships, punishment, rewards (Explain)

16. Nutrition — (24 hour recall including snacks)

Figure 13-3d

Pre-Pregnant Weight _____ Date _____ Pre-Pregnant BP _____ Date _____

MONITORING — COUNSELING

DATE	WT.	B.P.	VISITS WITH SCHOOL NURSE — COMMENTS: Inquire specifically re: nutrition, headache, altered vision, abdominal pain, nausea, vomiting, bleeding, fluid or secretions from vagina, dysuria. Comment about health, nutrition, any classes re: labor, delivery, etc. being taken by student.	LEARNING MODULE

Figure 13-4

LEADING CAUSES OF DEATH FOR U.S. MALES
15–34 YEARS (1991)*

Cause	Number	(%)
Accidents	23,108	(32)
Homicide	13,122	(18)
Suicide	9,434	(13)
HIV	8,661	(12)
Cancer	3,699	(5)
Other	13,234	(19)
	71,258	(100)

*Morbidity and Mortality Weekly Report 43 (40): 725–730, 1994.

Figure 13-5

RESOLUTION
CORPORAL PUNISHMENT IN THE SCHOOLS

WHEREAS   the National Association of School Nurses believes that all children have the right to education in a safe environment, free from physical harm; and

WHEREAS   school nurses, school administrators, school counselors, teachers and all other school personnel are responsible to report suspicion of child abuse;

THEREFORE, BE IT RESOLVED   that the National Association of School Nurses believes that corporal punishment should be abolished in all schools.

National Association of School Nurses

Adopted June 1989

CHAPTER 14

SCHOOL HEALTH: THE NEXT DECADE

Health Care Reform
Educational Restructuring
Computers and Other Technology
Nursing and School Nursing
New Diseases-Old Diseases
Research and Medical Trends
Community-School Partnerships
Summary
References
Chapter 14 Figures:

Chapter 14

SCHOOL HEALTH: THE NEXT DECADE

> If anyone had told me what wonderful changes
> were to take place here in 10 years, I wouldn't
> have believed it.
>
> *Mrs. Jo, in* Jo's Boys
> *Louisa May Alcott*

This chapter is not about what is, but what might be. Future school health services and the role of the school nurse will evolve out of a synthesis of national health care reform and educational restructuring. The possible combinations and permutations are numerous. I will attempt to project (not necessarily predict) a beneficial working model of school health based on current trends in health care and education. You are at the center, linking not only health and education but public and private sectors of society—a large and important role.

HEALTH CARE REFORM

While President Clinton's Health Security Plan did not pass during the 1994 congressional session, there was no substantive opposition to the concept of universal health coverage. There seemed to be unspoken agreement that health care was, perhaps, a right of citizenship; the debate centered around issues of definition and implementation.

What Is Universal Coverage?

The term, universal coverage, refers to some form of national health insurance for all citizens—cradle to grave. It would comprise a comprehensive package of core benefits. What is core and what ancillary is still being debated.

Another appealing element that met little opposition was portability: the coverage should move with the individual from place to place or job to job.

Who Will Pay for It?

The big four revenue sources being considered, and likely to be important in whatever bill is passed are

- employers
- employees
- budget cuts
- special sales taxes (cigarettes, etc.)

Measures to control costs will need to be carefully addressed. Certainly the cost of health care is not the result of forces beyond our control, but previous attempts at control have not worked consistently. Private insurance companies with their elaborate infrastructures will be prime targets in future cost containment. It is likely that some combination of competition and regulatory mechanisms will result. Administrative costs and duplication will also need to be curtailed.

How Will Delivery Be Affected?

While universal health coverage will be a national program, states will undoubtedly have options. A pure free-market system has not provided equal access, affordability, or portability. It will be up to the states to devise delivery systems within federal guidelines that meet the needs of their citizenry. Just how much flexibility they will have is unclear. It does seem certain that universal access, portability, quality, and cost-effectiveness will be key parameters monitored by Uncle Sam.

Decreasing duplicative efforts of multiple agencies will be critical to achieving cost-effectiveness. In turn, eliminating duplication will require health centers to house multiple services. In the case of school-aged students (and probably their families), it will surely mean more school-based and school-linked services; that's where the customers are. Sutton's Law: (When asked why he robbed banks, Willie Sutton replied, "Because that's where the money is.").

School-Based and School-Linked Services

Since families are the basic unit of society, and schools are the most ubiquitous institution in communities, it is inevitable that families and schools will be drawn closer together in more than educational pursuits. The integrated services concept can most easily be effected within the existing infrastructure of schools. School-based clinics have been the first step. As past ANA president, Lucille Joel, says: "Linking primary health care services for children to the school is just common sense, like linking health care benefits to the work place."

While school-based clinics have had a significant measure of success in most states, adding services and agencies (mental health, social service, etc.) is a monumental undertaking that will not happen overnight—even if consensus is reached that it should happen. See the section, "Community-School Partnerships" at the end of the chapter.

EDUCATIONAL RESTRUCTURING

Being part of the "education establishment," I see three weaknesses that require rectifying: (1) a tendency toward fads, (2) change for change's sake, and (3) a paucity of sound research and evaluation of methods and services. The health professions, especially school nurses who have established credibility, can exert a powerful influence on these weaknesses. When a new idea or model surfaces, ask, "How will this enhance student success?" Explore the literature and what has been done before. If there is a rational basis for trying something new, make sure to have an objective evaluation of the results by a disinterested party (implementers always believe they are successful because of ego involvement).

Current trends and elements that bear monitoring include

- changing student demographics
- changing family and social values
- research in the causes of underachievement and dropout
- computer-assisted instruction (and other technology)
- global economics and other work force issues (where will the jobs be?)
- shifting patterns of morbidity and mortality
- public policy (and public sentiment) for education
- educational restructuring
- alternative certification for teachers

Several of these bear further comment.

Tomorrow's Students

The children will be more challenging as they have more complicated problems at home. The trend toward more minority students will continue as will an increase in the number of students in lower socioeconomic levels and those speaking a variety of languages. These parameters carry with them the threat of inadequate health coverage—national health insurance notwithstanding—thus, a greater need for school-based health services. We will see an increasing number of disabled children as medical advances save more high-risk newborns, and consequently more students in schools with assistive devices.

Restructuring Schools

Under the umbrella of "restructuring" are a number of paradigms designed to rearrange the school's resources to better meet student needs. Included are such recent concepts as site-based management (more local autonomy with parent involvement), year-round school, education vouchers, charter schools, and privatization.

Under the voucher system, dollars follow the student to the school of choice. Charter schools allow individuals (parents among them) or existing schools to apply to their state education department for special waivers to "do their own thing" (as long as student performance meets certain standards). Michigan is currently leading the nation in this effort: One example is the Northlane Math and Science Academy. Privatization means asking a private firm to run the school. Baltimore was the first large urban district to attempt this on a large scale.

What all these attempts at restructuring tell us is that the uniformity of school systems, once thought to be a virtue, is clearly a liability in the modern era.

Year-round schools seem to be catching on more rapidly than other restructuring efforts. Why? From the pedagogical standpoint, the justification is that much learning is lost during the summer. An increasing number of studies support the contention that interspersing frequent short vacations is more educationally sound. As well, with one-fourth to one-third of students off at any given time, space, supply, and transportation needs are less although actual cost savings have not been documented yet.

Alternative Certification for Teachers

A shortage of quality teacher applicants in specific subject areas has stimulated some communities to look to alternative methods of certifying teachers (rather than a college degree in education); math, science, and foreign language are examples. The process involves hiring individuals from private industry and training them to function in the classroom. To date, some success has been achieved through these efforts.

A related concept is "grow your own." Some districts are paying part of college education costs for graduating seniors who agree to come back to teach in the district. The jury is still out on this one.

Educational Research

A greater emphasis will be placed on scientific evaluation of effective teaching methods. Currently, techniques used with hearing impaired students (signing and lipreading) show promise for helping students with learning disabilties and normal hearing.

COMPUTERS AND OTHER TECHNOLOGY

Metallic wizardry is all the rage. It is amazing, mystical, and fun, but what are the real advantages of computers? There are only two: speed and accuracy. School districts, notorious for their multitude of report forms (daily, weekly, monthly, 6-weekly, semester/semiannual, annual) are computerizing in droves. Now that computerization of administrative functions is well under way, schools are seriously looking at and piloting additional uses of technology in education. One of the most promising is computer assisted instruction (CAI).

Computer-Assisted Instruction

Research has amply demonstrated that educational technology has a significant positive effect on student achievement; students feel more successful in school, are more motivated to learn, and have increased confidence when they use computer-based instruction. CAI allows students to move at their own pace and receive immediate feedback for their responses. This frees teachers to provide more individual help to students having difficulty, rather than conduct lock-step activities.

If CAI is so great, why has its implementation been slow in most schools? Three reasons account for most of the explanation:

- initial cost of hardware for every classroom
- inadequate teacher training
- limited software programs to fit the curriculum

The first problem is being solved by multiyear phase-in budgeting. The second problem, teacher training, has three elements: teacher acceptance, computer literacy, and ability to select software programs that piggyback and reinforce the existing curriculum. It requires time and money to train teachers, and appropriate trainers are scarce in many areas. The third barrier, limited software programs, is a problem primarily because the educational product was not as profitable as business software. This situation has been much improved by book publishers' subsidizing software development firms and by expansion of the market; more schools have computers now and parents are buying educational software. Look for an explosion of CAI in the classroom over the next few years.

The Computerized School Clinic

Bergren's overview of this subject appeared in the *Journal of School Nursing* (1993). Bergren recommends a three-step process for computerizing a school clinic:

- Identify specific needs and goals (start with existing forms and reports).
- Select software, or programs to meet those needs (some prepackaged programs for student health records are Dynomite and Health Master).
- Choose the hardware required to run the software.

Many people attack the issue in reverse order and wind up with less than they had hoped for; some become frustrated and abandon computerization. Keep in mind that computers don't think; they do only what humans tell (program) them to do. It takes a lot of thought and preparation to come up with an efficient system.

An alternative approach to step 2 (selecting software) is especially applicable if your school district has or is planning a systemwide integrated computer network (usually a central mainframe with peripheral connections to each local campus). These "umbrella networks" are custom designed, or at least modified, to fit the needs of a particular school system. If you have such a network, you will want your clinic computer to access the central mainframe, or at least the campuswide student data base. That way you can create your own health files from existing student demographic data; otherwise you will have to enter all names, addresses, birthdates, and grades—basic data for each student. Once you have this linkage, you can tell the district computer consultant or programmer what health data you will need space for. To determine space needed, combine current manually collected data and review commercial student health records software. Most companies, for example Dynomite and Health Master, have free demonstration disks.

It is wise to pilot at least two campuses before deciding to go districtwide. Visiting a school nurse who is already using a computerized system is invaluable.

Other Technologies

Technocrats on the cutting edge estimate that half the technology we will be using by the millennium hasn't even been invented! New computer technology, on average, becomes obsolete after 90 days on the market. Frequent upgrades are a must.

In addition to computerizing student health records (spreadsheet and data base functions), the word processing function saves time by printing various predetermined parent letters and standard student care plans.

Various communication links speed transfer of information, for instance:

- receive records from other sites
- send records
- send and receive electronic mail
- FAX information (modem with dedicated telephone line required)
- access Internet for multiple services and information
- electronic claims processing (Medicaid)
- physician consultation to remote sites

Still other capabilities include computerized

- medical dictionary and spell checker
- *Physicians Desk Reference (PDR)*
- scanning and storage of forms, letters and other documents (avoids paper files)
- statistical analyses (calculate the average blood pressure of 8th grade females)
- instruction for staff and students (anatomy, etc.)
- literature searches (through Medline, ERIC, Psychological Abstracts, and other databases)
- graphics

Ultimately, diagnosis and treatment will be facilitated by computer: Key in the patient's symptoms and receive a list of differential diagnoses in decreasing order of probability with recommended treatment or further tests. One such fledgling program already exists: Iliad for PC or Macintosh (1-800-832-1000), which contains 11,910 disease manifestations. It can also be used as an electronic research library to review specific diseases or test your skills in clinical problem solving through simulated patient cases.

Journals and review courses are also available on CD-ROM (compact disk-read only memory). To view these, your computer will need a CD-ROM drive for about $200. The "read only" means you cannot add to or delete from the laser disk as you can using a standard 3½" square floppy disk. CD-ROM disks also have the capability for motion and sound. Videodiscs are large (not compact) and used by libraries. The multimedia capabilities of video discs will increase their popularity as prices fall.

Security and Confidentiality

Since all student health information is confidential, computer security is an important consideration. Most systems rely on passwords to access specific data. Multiple passwords, keyed in to a program, can limit access to various levels. For instance, you may want to allow teacher access to demographic, immunization, and screening data, but not to medical diagnoses or progress notes. Their password allows them limited entry, while yours gives you full access.

Information stored in a computer is more secure than that stored in paper files, yet hard copies can be printed when needed. We are getting closer to the paperless clinic, but don't forget back-up disks for important data. All computers "crash" eventually—lightning storms and other causes of power surges are especially treacherous.

NURSING AND SCHOOL NURSING

National nursing leadership is predicting that the next decade will see a continued shift of hospital nurses into the community (in 1994, 40% of hospital beds were unoccupied). For those nurses relocated into the community, there will also be a shift away from specialization.

Many possibilities exist for the location and nature of increased community health services. Existing health centers and hospital satellite clinics are prime locations for expansion. Itinerant services and other "clinics without walls" will proliferate. School sites will be considered more closely. We will probably see an increase in independent nurse practice, the extent of which will hinge on states' granting nurses independent prescriptive authority and insurance companies' willingness to pay nurses directly. Many states currently provide for independent nurse practice in rural areas, so it would be a logical step to expand this to additional underserved areas, such as the inner city. Increased malpractice risk for nurses will certainly be an issue.

A shift to community-based practice for nurses will require significant educational efforts to retool the specialist, such as an ICU nurse, into the comprehensive generalist. Schools of nursing will play a key role.

As more health services are offered in schools, proactive school nurses will assume increasingly important roles in triage, case management, and coordination. At last survey (Igoe 1994), there were 30,979 school nurses in the 50 states, with no shortage of applicants. These numbers will expand along with the number of health services simply because any school or school system that sees its roles as supporting a student's ability to learn is a potential base for a full range of primary health services delivered by advance-practice nurses.

School nurses understand that the best way to increase accessibility of services to children is to go to them. Continuity of care, so important to quality, is built in to schools; consistent, known providers are more likely to obtain good results. The school setting is also a natural site to accommodate the greater emphasis on prevention and wellness because of existing health education classes and health counseling by school nurses.

Two barriers to rapid expansion of school health services are finances and philosophy. With regard to the latter, some health institutions are not eager to acknowledge schools as appropriate sites for primary health care. Some schools do not relish the responsibility and its accompanying theoretical increase in liability. This philosophical resistance will diminish as more expanded school health models demonstrate success. In the last section of this chapter, we will look at community linkages that show promise for speeding the expansion of health care for students and their families.

The other barrier, finances, is more perceived than real. Dollars already exist from multiple programs, both educational (Chapter 1) and medical (Medicaid), which, if rechanneled, could finance expanded school health services.

Good advice to school nurses who wish to influence this process and their own future comes from Marla Salmon (see references). She says, in paraphrase,

> Moving forward means abandoning old ways of seeing and doing things. With the increasing interest in school-linked health services, national health insurance, etc., it is timely for the nursing establishment to formulate its positions and begin presenting them to the public.
>   Because of the variety of practice models for school nursing, it is unlikely that total consensus will be achieved within the profession. But it is essential that there be agreement on core elements before splinter groups give the impression of disunity.

The first step toward unity is a further shift toward disease prevention and health promotion. The increasing recognition of school-based clinics and nurse practitioners should also be factored into the process, as they will most surely increase with or without input from the school nursing profession.

After establishment of common ground within the profession, it is then necessary to identify leaders who can represent these "inside" nursing issues to the "outside" in a manner that demonstrates unity. While national health care reform is developing, many state and local reforms are already underway. This makes it important that school nurses move rapidly to help steer these activities in the right direction. If they do not join the process, the school nurses' role will be created for them.

When it comes to school health services, it is time for nurses to ask, "Who is making the decisions?" School nurses have good credibility, but sometimes they hesitate to involve themselves in the messy process necessary to effect social change (political and otherwise). Now is not the time to be timid.

NEW DISEASES-OLD DISEASES

Infections

A few short years ago, we thought that infectious diseases would soon be extinct. The eradication of smallpox and decline of polio and other vaccine-preventable diseases lulled us into complacency. David R. Smith, the Texas Commissioner of Health in 1994 said

> Busy parents let immunization schedules slide. Health professionals turned their attention to chronic illnesses such as cancer and heart disease. Taxpayers and elected officials shifted their priorities from disease prevention to crime and other concerns.

Public health watchdogs were called off—so our early warning system of disease surveillance is not up to speed. Laboratories were allowed to languish—so our ability to identify and respond quickly to disease threats is compromised.

We have been recently shocked and unprepared to protect ourselves adequately from reemerging disease such as tuberculosis, much less from newly emerging threats like Lyme disease, E. coli, hantavirus, or necrotizing fasciitis.

Antibiotics, the "miracle drugs" against infectious diseases, have been overused so that some disease-causing organisms, such as tuberculosis and gonorrhea, have become resistant. Even common childhood ear infections have become more difficult to cure.

Infectious diseases remain the leading cause of death worldwide. In the United States HIV infection, pneumonia, and influenza are among the top 10 killers.

The following highlights of selected diseases provide an overview of infectious challenges. (Source: *Morbidity and Mortality Weekly Report*, U.S. Public Health Service, October, 1994.)

- *Lyme Disease*—this tick-borne spirochetal disease, while not increasing rapidly, is still difficult to diagnose for those who have no experience with it. The largest number of cases are found on the Atlantic coast, in the upper Midwest and in the West. There is no evidence of person-to-person transmission. Serologic tests are negative early in the disease and often in those treated with antibiotics. Treatment is with tetracycline for adults and amoxicillin for children.

- *E. Coli Bacteria*—In 1993, an outbreak of *E. coli* O 157 affected more than 500 people in four western states, resulting in 56 cases of hemolytic uremic syndrome and four deaths. Because of this outbreak, many clinical laboratories began screening stool samples for *E. coli* O 157, which resulted in the identification of many more cases. In May 1993, the Council of State and Territorial Epidemiologists (CSTE) passed a resolution recommending that *E. coli* O 157 infection be made reportable by all states and territories.

- *Hantavirus*—Hantavirus Pulmonary Syndrome (HPS), a newly recognized illness characterized by an influenzalike prodrome followed by the acute onset of respiratory failure, was first identified in the southwestern United States in June 1993 during the investigation of a cluster of unexplained deaths. A new hantavirus (Sin Nombre virus) and a rodent reservoir for the virus (the deer mouse [Peromyscus maniculatus]) were identified. As of August, 1994, national surveillance for HPS, initiated by CDC in coordination with CSTE, has identified 91 confirmed cases of HPS (with 48 deaths) in 20 states (case fatality rate: 53%).

- *Necrotizing Fasciitis*—During 1993, CDC surveillance for invasive group A streptococcal infections (necrotizing fasciitis) consisted of a passive nationwide surveillance system. This system operated through the collection of isolates from normally sterile sites and the collection of case reports. Although current data on incidence and trends for invasive disease, streptococcal toxic shock syndrome, and necrotizing fasciitis are not available, population-based active surveillance for these infections has begun in several geographic areas and was expanded in 1994 as part of surveillance for emerging infectious diseases.

- *Pneumococcus*—The increasing incidence of drug-resistant *Streptococcus pneumoniae (pneummococcus)* strains in the United States has created an emerging public health challenge. CDC surveillance data from 1992 indicated that the prevalence of pneumococcal strains that are highly resistant to penicillin increased 60-fold (from 0.02% to 1.3%) when compared with the prevalence of isolates collected from 1979 through 1987. CDC and CSTE are developing better surveillance techniques for 1995 and beyond.

- *Tuberculosis*—Between 1992 and 1993, the number of reported tuberculosis cases in the United States decreased from 26,673 to 25,313. This decrease may be associated with the effectiveness of prevention and control measures implemented during the period 1989–1993. However, two other factors also may be responsible for the decrease, including (1) delayed reporting caused by use of a new CDC tuberculosis reporting form and the change from paper records to a computerized system, and (2) underreporting because of modification of the AIDS case definition. Most alarming is the emergence of a multidrug-resistant strain of the tubercle bacillus.

- *AIDS*—In 1993, the number of AIDS cases reported to CDC increased 127% from the number reported in 1992. The large increase in the number of cases was largely due to changes in the 1993 AIDS case definition. As of January 1, 1993, HIV-infected persons with additional clinical conditions, as well as those with markers of severe immunosuppression, were defined as having AIDS.

- *Hepatitis B*—The reported incidence of hepatitis B decreased 59% from 1985 through 1993. This decline was caused by decreases in the number of cases reported among homosexual men between 1985 and 1989 and in the number reported among injecting-drug users from 1989 through 1992. These decreases are thought to result from an increase in AIDS awareness, which has resulted in behavioral changes (e.g., safer sex and needle-using practices). Adolescents are the new target for hepatitis B prevention with vaccine being recommended for those at risk (primarily those who are sexually active). Newborns are receiving the vaccine in many areas.

- *Haemophilus influenzae*—The rate of *Haemophilus influenzae* disease as reported through the National Notifiable Diseases Surveillance System (NNDSS) has continued to decline. Rates decreased 95% between 1987 and 1993. Data collected by active surveillance from selected sites indicate that the decline is primarily in *Haemophilus influenzae* type b (Hib) disease among children < 5 years of age. This decline is associated with the use of the newly licensed Hib conjugate vaccines.

- *Sexually Transmitted Diseases*—Nationally, the rates for gonorrhea and primary and secondary syphilis have declined since 1990, reaching low points in 1993 that were below or approaching the Year 2000 Objectives (≤225 cases gonorrhea and ≤10 cases primary and secondary syphilis per 100,000 persons). However, rates for both diseases remained higher than the Year 2000 Objectives for certain population subgroups: adolescents and young adults, minorities (especially African Americans), and persons living in the southern United States.

Because of the ability of viruses and bacteria to mutate, we will continue to see emerging and changing diseases as well as shifting antibiotic resistance. In fact, a whole new class of drugs must be developed to stay ahead of the growing legions of drug-resistant bacteria. There are some new agents being developed by pharmaceutical houses that will be useful in the future, but are not available yet.

One way to prevent resistance problems is to use antibiotics in a more restrained fashion. Physicians are often guilty of succumbing to patient pressure to prescribe antibiotics for colds—which, of course, have no value unless secondary infection occurs. The "prophylactic" use of antibiotics is an important cause of bacterial resistance.

Currently, for some organisms, there are no new antibiotics to turn to. For the first time in a long while, we are not able to treat certain organisms very effectively.

In 1995, a nationwide surveillance network was established to track potentially lethal antibiotic resistant pathogens in hospitals and medical centers throughout the United States. The project acronym is SCOPE (*S*urveillance and *C*ontrol of *P*athogens of *E*pidemiologic importance) and will be overseen by the University of Iowa School of Medicine.

Environmental Issues

As our society becomes more advanced, it becomes, at the same time, safer *and* more dangerous. Is that statement oxymoronic?

No, it simply means there are trade-offs as science and technology advance. Chapter 10 provided an overview of current environmental hazards in the school setting. "Sick building syndrome" is one of our more recent challenges, although medical feedback to architects and builders has resulted in improved building construction with better ventilation.

Chemical sensitivities are a group of clinical syndromes beginning to surface. In fact, "multiple chemical sensitivities" is a diagnosis cropping up more frequently. Whether this entity has a purely physiological basis or is psychogenic remains to be seen. Three pieces of evidence suggest the latter: (1) only chemicals with significant odors seem to trigger symptoms, (2) none of the symptoms are documentable (headache, dizziness, etc.), and (3) many of the individuals affected have mental health diagnoses (such as depression or bipolar disorder). While this confusion will be sorted out in time, each school system must have a plan for dealing with this medical diagnosis. There will be Workers' Compensation issues to grapple with.

Employee Mental Health

It is likely that emotional problems will become one of the areas of greatest concern in the next decade. Work-related stress seems to be increasing in both private industry and the public sector; schools are no exception: The pressure to improve student achievement is great.

What is the primary source?

Job-induced stress may be caused by either internal thoughts ("I may lose my job") or conflicts (whether to report a violation of safety code) or external factors such as supervisors, co-workers, or events (downsizing) in the workplace.

For some employees, stress may be cumulative, becoming the proverbial "straw that breaks the camel's back." For others, excessive stress may have sudden onset as a reaction to a physical injury. Depending upon the job skills required, a person can work with any number of physical injuries, yet *all jobs require a mind*. When the mind is seriously compromised because of stress—when memory, concentration, and attention are impaired—the person cannot function as effectively.

Unfortunately, most symptoms of stress are invisible and few can be measured in a laboratory setting. As such, the symptoms of stress can be faked, which leads to skepticism and disbelief among employers, family members, and even sufferers that the symptoms are truly evidence of serious psychological distress.

The six most common work situations leading to disabling stress are

- a physical injury on the job resulting in job loss
- a traumatic event on the job, such as a robbery or assault
- a dysfunctional supervisor
- scapegoating by peers
- sexual harassment
- unethical or illegal activity

Stress reduction programs are merely bandaids when the primary source is unaltered.

Managers, while they should expect their directives to be carried out, need to be cognizant of how they issue them, and how they treat their employees in general. Every employee can and should be treated fairly and with respect. Directives are equally binding whether whispered or shouted. Managers of the future will need to pay more attention to the mental hygiene of their subordinates—if they want to be perceived as effective managers.

RESEARCH AND MEDICAL TRENDS

The following kaleidoscope of major trends will help you visualize the potential impact on your practice and your clients:

Respiratory Care

Respiratory dependent premature infants will be weaned more easily, facilitating school attendance.

Tuberculosis will continue to increase, including drug-resistant strains.

By the year 2000, the climbing death rate for asthma will be reversed by more extensive monitoring with peak flow meters and greater use of inhaled steroids, such as beclomethazone (Beclovent inhaler).

Neurosciences

Cochlear implants for the treatment of nerve deafness will increase. The best hearing and speech results to date have been seen in three- to five-year-olds who had acquired deafness (as from meningitis or mumps) after some speech has developed.

A new class of anticonvulsants that have a more focused and localized action on epileptigenic neurons in the brain will be developed. They will be more effective and have fewer motor and cognitive side effects.

A refinement in the treatment of brain tumors with stereotactic laser surgery will allow for removal of formerly inoperable growths—all without injuring surrounding tissue.

Advances will be seen in the discovery of genetic markers for neurodegenerative diseases. Markers for Huntington's disease and Alzheimer's have already been found. Better genetic counseling of parents with one affected child will be available.

Research is also underway to evaluate the efficacy of biofeedback in the treatment of attention deficit hyperactivity disorder.

Cancer

Earlier diagnosis and resulting better prognosis will stem from laboratory tests that identify tumor markers in the bloodstream. Already in use are prostate-specific antigen (PSA) and cancer antigen-125 for ovarian cancer.

The logical next step after early diagnosis is more effective treatment for cancer. This will likely result from the refinement of monoclonal antibodies—antitumor substances produced by injecting mice with human tumor cells. This kind of treatment is more focused, since these antibodies will attack only cancer cells, not normal ones.

The future also promises more than new treatments for cancer. Lifestyle changes will make people healthier and less cancer prone. The evidence is mounting that diet and exercise do affect many cancers. A positive effect is being reported by Kenneth Cooper (the aerobics man) with moderate exercise (too much actually has a negative effect), a balanced, high-fiber diet, and three specific vitamins: C, E, and beta-carotene.

Immunology

Better ways to both suppress and stimulate the immune system will be discovered. Tacrolimus (previously called FK 506) was approved by the FDA in 1994 for primary prevention of organ rejection in patients receiving liver transplants. Additional good news for children needing liver transplants is the perfection of the technique of living related-donor transplants. A living relative, who is found to be tissue compatible, donates a portion of the left lobe of his or her liver. This can be done before the child's health deteriorates.

Techniques for stimulating the immune system, in children who are born deficient or individuals with AIDS or other immune-suppressing disorders, will probably evolve from research on a newly discovered regulatory gene that governs the formation of lymphocytes and other cells in the immune system. Researchers at the University of Chicago have described a mouse gene for transcription factor PU-1; mice lacking it all die due to the lack of all immune cells. Theoretically, a similar factor in humans could stimulate the production of immune cells.

Biotechnology

The fastest growing and most controversial area of scientific research is the collaboration between universities and private industry. Universities need money and private biotechnology industries (such as pharmaceutical houses) need scientists, so many such marriages have occurred throughout the country.

Biology became big business in 1973 when Cohen and Boyer invented a technique that made genetic engineering practical. They worked out a way to transplant functioning genes from different organisms into bacteria, which could then be grown in large quantities and made into minifactories, producing the protein directed by the inserted gene. Voila—a cost effective way to produce therapeutic substances!

At the beginning of 1995, there were 1300 biotechnology firms in the United States. In 1989, this industry overtook government as the primary financial provider for biomedical research, after decades of federal dominance. The result is that universities, no longer certain of federal support for basic research, have started courting the private sector. Most of the results have been good; that is, useful products have reached the marketplace faster. The only concern is that the big leaps in science usually happen when good scientists are allowed to follow their imaginations—not pragmatic, short term goals.

Examples of the fruitfulness of these marriages between academia and industry include the production of human insulin synthetically, as well as interferon and the hepatitis B vaccine.

New Medications and Routes of Administration

Iontophoresis—the process by which medication patches infuse drugs through the skin—will expand. Common drugs administered in patches in 1995 are scopolamine (motion sickness), estradiol (menopause), and nicotine (for smoking cessation).

More drugs will be given nasally. At present, the most dramatic and effective example is antidiuretic hormone (ADH) for diabetes insipidus.

Microinfusers to deliver insulin through the skin are currently being tested.

A new class of compounds that inhibit the ability of a virus to assemble into an infectious particle is being studied in several laboratories.

Gizmos and Gadgets

The broad field of telecommunications will experience a second phase explosion, with all manner of devices to monitor individual patients by phone or satellite linkage (telemetry)—for instance, cardiac rhythm in a patient prone to ventricular tachycardia. The same patient could also have a microcardioverter implanted to kick in when a predetermined heart rate is reached on the monitor.

Professional and Paraprofessional Roles

While many of the predicted advances will make health care delivery to the individual more effective and efficient, there will not be enough health professionals to go around if some form of universal health coverage passes Congress. More tasks will be delegated to paraprofessionals, and longer waits for care will surely result initially. Increased delegation will produce ethical and legal concerns from nurses and others. Civil liability and malpractice judgments will increase unless health professionals provide for a smooth transition to greater involvement of nurse aides and others through quality training and monitoring.

COMMUNITY-SCHOOL PARTNERSHIPS

Do We Need Them?

The answer is a resounding yes, except possibly in the most affluent communities. A partnership allows local communities to deal with issues beyond the resources of individual agencies; pooled resources are greater than the sum of the parts in providing a greater benefit to clients.

While student health needs are increasing in number and complexity, basic health and social services remain fragmented, inaccesible, or simply unavailable. We clearly need comprehensive, integrated service delivery approaches that are communitywide and coordinate various services—including education, health, social service, and family support.

Ninety-five percent of the 55 million children in the United States, ages 5 to 18, attend school. Therefore, school is the logical choice for health resources that espouse illness prevention and wellness promotion. Neither schools nor agencies are providing comprehensive health care for children. It's time to stop pigeonholing diseases and dollars and begin to look at seamless service; society bears some responsibility for helping parents and family members meet their own needs.

Which Models Work Best?

Movers and shakers who have developed school-community partnerships have come to the same conclusion: Each community must develop its own approach to cooperation and integrated services based on local needs. There are, however, certain basics that apply to every community. These include performing a needs assessment, and having clearly defined goals, a budget, role descriptions, and a governance structure.

One of the first decisions to be made is where to locate the clinic: within a school building, on a school campus, or at a community site. In some communities, linking schools to a community-based model may be preferable or more acceptable than housing such services in schools. Experience, however, has shown that using the infrastructure of public schools permits delivery of a wide spectrum of primary health care that is both cost-effective and equitably distributed throughout a community. In addition, the percentage of students participating is higher when the facility is on campus, presumably due to the increased accessibility and easier coordination with school officials. Since parent involvement is essential to success, the schools also provide a familiar location that is comfortable; parents already have rapport with the school staff. Interestingly, there is no significant relationship between the size of the city and the extent of school-based health services on the national scene.

The goal, from the educator's standpoint, is to decrease out-of-class time, which means decreasing out-of-school referrals. School systems do not always easily accommodate the values and styles of operation of the health care system; however, once services begin, educators seem to undergo a mental adjustment that causes them to be great supporters of the services. The greatest usage of school-based clinics is seen at the middle school level, which confirms both educators' and health professionals' experience that early adolescence is the time of greatest turmoil.

Predetermined models cannot be superimposed *in toto* on any community; however, some general models provide a starting point for planning. One is the separate clinic building on the school campus. This is the most expensive model and perhaps the ideal. It has all the advantages of being on campus and accessible to students with none of the disadvantages of being inside the building. In this case, the clinic staff, who may be from the county hospital, health department, or a nursing school, may maintain their distance and autonomy as a separate entity and not become involved with the details of school procedures.

A second model, which is probably the most cost-effective and easiest to implement, is the visiting team. An itinerant health team usually consists of a nurse practitioner or physician assistant, a social worker, and a paraprofessional who doubles as a medical assistant and clerk. The team has telephone consultation and occasional onsite visits with a pediatrician or adolescent specialist. The cost of this team varies, depending on salaries, but runs from $110,000 to $125,000 per year.

Regardless of which model is chosen, it is important to ensure that you, as the school nurse, are carefully integrated into the system. Generally, you should be the referral originator to the school-based clinic and the case manager for the students you refer—the hub of the wheel. Of course, students can refer themselves and parents may refer their children directly to the clinic without your knowledge; however, over the long haul, most referrals come from you.

Integration of social, mental health, and medical services acknowledges the complex causes of many of the problems of today's youth. As Dr. Sidney Gellis said of one Canadian school-based clinic: "It seems logical that schools should become the physical location for multi-disciplinary health care covering many aspects of physical, emotional, educational, and social health. Teachers, pediatricians, parents, psychiatrists, and children can move mountains if they work together under the same roof rather than writing each other letters and faxing lengthy reports."

How Do You Create Them?

Once the decision has been made to locate the clinic in one of three places (off campus, on campus in a separate building, or within the school building), you then begin a needs assessment: a survey of the consumers to determine what services are to be offered (see Chapter 1). The essential steps in promoting a community-school health partnership are:

- Create a community vision.
- Define partnership parameters.
- Identify barriers.
- Agree on goals (include all stakeholders, especially parents and students).
- Examine models.
- Develop trust (allow time).
- Identify funding sources.
- Implement a pilot model.
- Evaluate and revise.
- Implement a schoolwide program.

Figure 14-1, at the end of this chapter, lists the essentials of service integration for school- or community-based clinics. The leadership element is most important and generally should be shared among agencies. If two major agencies are participating, there should be co-chairs; if there are three or more, form a board or other mechanism for shared decision making.

Figure 14-2 lists possible agency sponsors. It also indicates sources of financial support customarily utilized. Collaborators should be equal partners and formal partnerships must be flexible and responsive to new insights to problems. To achieve true collaboration, many people must be empowered with decision-making capabilities.

What are some of the obstacles to developing functioning school-community partnerships? They are the same that we encounter in any project where two or more agencies are attempting to collaborate:

- Differences in philosophy—Many agencies have a narrow focus in terms of their delivery system. They may focus on one physical illness or only on mental illness, with a limited ability to consider a holistic approach; they generally have budget constraints because of specific criteria for serving their clients.
- Territory and control.
- Funding.
- Accessibility (weekends and summer).
- Lack of unanimous community support.

Individuals who have specific agendas (and often do not have children in the school system) may use misinformation to try to cause a project to fail; they may refer to the school-based clinic as a birth control clinic or abortion clinic. The best defense is to have public hearings before either a board of education or some other body to allow people to speak and to present information. Most school-based clinics report that approximately 85% of their visits are for comprehensive health care and 15% for family planning counseling.

A key point in the creation of acceptable and effective school- or community-based health services is the need to ensure consumer choice. Parents are responsible for making health choices for their children. Figure 14-3 is an example of a consent form that provides a menu of services from which parents or guardians may choose. It is structured so that specific services *not* desired are circled. If parents do *not* wish their child to receive family planning counseling, they circle item 7. The permission form should be signed annually by a parent. As students enter the secondary level, they participate in the decision making to an increasing degree and self-referral to the clinic (after initial parent permission) becomes more common. One point that varies from state to state is the age at which certain problems may be treated by professionals without parent notification (for example, sexually transmitted diseases).

How Do You Sustain Them?

Even the most carefully designed program will fail if funding is not sustained. Grants and private sector funds rarely provide stable funding. Federal categorical funding is exceedingly complex and contains strict eligibility criteria. Decentralization of selected federal programs would bring greater cohesion and flexibility to services for children and families.

There is no sure solution to funding problems, but the goal must be to secure a reliable, continuing source. In some communities county hospital districts have established satellite clinics, which they see as the wave of the future. These satellites can be located on school campuses, and county tax dollars can become a continuing source of funding. Local health departments and state health departments are another source because of their commitment to prevention. Schools have been known to build the clinics to house outside health professionals (after a change in mind-set regarding the school's "responsibility").

Those who become discouraged in getting a project off the ground or in sustaining it will be energized by the comment of Dr. Robert Bruininks, Dean of the College of Education at the University of Minnesota.

> Our failure to act today will only defer to the next generation the rising social, moral, and financial costs of our neglect. Investing in our children is no longer a luxury but a national imperative.

SUMMARY

Changes in health care delivery and educational restructuring are setting the stage for ever increasing school-community linkages. Whatever the nature of these changes may be, whatever new pathologies and technologies arise, there will always be a need for the human to human contact in securing and maintaining wellness. You provide that human element and cement the link between school and community, between health and education, and between public and private sectors of society.

While it is important to keep abreast of the latest trends, it is even better to anticipate and set trends. Don't plan your future like a pontoon bridge, each petty span no longer than its predecessor. The future belongs to the visionary and the brave.

REFERENCES

1. Bennett, R. "Questions to Ask Your Congressman About Health Care Reform." *Readers Digest,* August, 1994.

2. Bergren, M. "You Decide to Computerize, Now What?" *Journal of School Nursing* 9(4):26, 1993.

3. Bialo, E. *The Effectiveness of Technology in Schools.* New York: Interactive Educational Systems Design, 1994.

4. Bruininks, R. "Integrating Services: The Case for Better Links to Schools." *Journal of School Health* 64(6):242, 1994.

5. Doyle, D. "The Role of Private Sector Management in Public Education." *Phi Delta Kappan,* October, 1994.

6. Emmett, A. "Health Care Trends That Will Reshape Nursing." *Nursing 94,* April, 1994.

7. *Expanding School Health Services to Serve Familes in the 21st Century.* American Nurses Association, Kansas City, MO, 1994.

8. Gandara, P. Year-Round Schooling as an Avenue to Major Structural Reform." *Educational Evaluation and Policy Analysis* 16(1):67, 1994.

9. Hacker, K. "A Nationwide Survey of School Health Services Delivery in Urban Schools." *Journal of School Health* 64(7):279, 1994.

10. "Health Care Reform and the School Nurse." *NASN Newsletter* 9(1):1, 1994.

11. *The Health of Young People: A Challenge and a Promise.* Geneva: World Health Organization, 1993.

12. Igoe, J. *National Survey of School Nurses and School Nurse Supervisors.* Scarborough, ME: National Association of School Nurses, 1994.

13. Joel, L. "Closing the School Health Safety Net." *American Journal of Nursing,* September, 1994.

14. Kawamoto, K. "Nursing Leadership: To Thrive in a World of Change." *Nursing Administration Quarterly,* 18(3):1–6, 1994.

15. Klenow, C. "Teaching with Technology: Hands-On." *Instructor* 102(8):83, 1993.

16. Knollmueller, R. "Thinking About Tomorrow for Nursing." *Journal of Continuing Education for Nurses* 25(5):196, 1994.

17. Knox, G. "Seven Rules to Year-Round Schooling." *School Administrator* 51(3):22–24, 1994.

18. Kohles, M. "On the Move to the 21st Century." *Nursing Administration Quarterly* 16(1):22, 1991.

19. Lorie, P. *History of the Future,* New York: Doubleday, 1989.

20. Lowe, B. "Integrated School Health Services." *Pediatrics* 94(3):400, 1994.

21. Mossinghoff, G. *New Medicines in Development for Women.* Washington, DC: Pharmaceutical Research and Manufacturers of America, 1994.

22. Rienzo, B. "The Politics of School-Based Clinics: A Community-Level Analysis." *Journal of School Health* 63(6):266, 1993.

23. Salmon, M. "The Future of School Nursing." *Journal of School Health* 64(4):137, 1994.

24. Schuman, A. "New Technologies for Pediatrics—1994." *Contemporary Pediatrics* (Supplement: Pediatricians Procedure Guide) September, 1994.

25. Siri, D. "Community-School Partnerships: A Vision for the Future." In *The Comprehensive School Health Challenge—Promoting Health Through Education.* Scotts Valley, CA: ETR Associates, 1994.

26. Smith, D. "Who's Afraid of the Big Bad Wolf?" *Disease Prevention News* 54(22):6, 1994.

27. Stetson, D. "Computers as Clinical Consultants." *Contemporary Pediatrics* 11:53, 1994.

28. U.S. Public Health Service. *Healthy People 2000 Midcourse Revisions.* Washington, DC, 1994.

29. Wallis, C. "A Class of Their Own." *Time,* October 31, 1994. (Charter Schools)

30. Yates, S. "The Practice of School Nursing: Integration with New Models of Health Service Delivery." *Journal of School Nursing* 10(1):10, 1994.

Figure 14-1

ESSENTIALS OF SERVICE INTEGRATION FOR
SCHOOL- OR COMMUNITY-BASED CLINICS*

Leadership Behavior:
- role of integrator
- long-term commitment
- promote systemic thinking, shared vision, and team learning

Stakeholder's Values:
- responsive to consumer (holistic)
- standards for quality prevention and intervention that are client-responsive
- broad support for values by constituents (professionals, citizens, and communities)

Structure:
- uniform data bases and language across systems; uniform confidentiality regulations
- linkage modes for outreach, intake, diagnosis, referral, and follow-up services
- linkage for fiscal, planning and programming, personnel practices, and administrative support management
- policies and regulations that encourage collaborative decisions and behaviors.

Resources:
- reinvestment of existing resources, fiscal flexibility, incentive funding for pilots
- ongoing evaluation of results
- interprofessional education, investment in public awareness and public contribution

*Adapted from Bruininks, 1994.

Figure 14-2

SCHOOL-BASED CLINIC COMPONENTS

Possible Agency Sponsors (various combinations)

> School of Nursing
> Hospital
> Medical School
> Community-based Organization (profit and nonprofit)
> Public Health Department
> Community Health Clinic
> Mental Health Agency

Budget Support (including in-kind)

> Federal
> > EPSDT
> > SHARS (School Health & Related Services)[1]
> > Medicaid Administrative Claiming (MAC)[2]
> > Maternal & Child Health Block Grants
> > Title X
> > Title XX
> > Chapter One
>
> State
> > General Funds
> > Health Department
> > Human Services Department
> > Education Department
>
> County/City Government
> > Local School District
> > Client Fees
> > Private Insurance
> > Private Foundations
> > Community Health Centers

[1] Reimbursement to schools for services to Special Education students

[2] Reimbursement to schools for management/administrative activities on behalf of Medicaid-eligible students.

Figure 14-3

PEDIATRIC PRIMARY CARE CONSENT FORM

Patient's Name: _____ Sex: M ____ F ____

Medicaid Number: _____

Patient's Birthdate: _____ Parent/Guardian: _____

Home Address: _____ Telephone Number: _____

Patient Allergies: _____ Parent Work Number: _____

Dear Parent or Guardian:

The XYZ Clinic provides adolescent health care services. It is necessary for you to sign this form for your child to receive health care. The following services are available:

1. First Aid and Minor Emergency Care
2. Well Check-ups and Annual Physicals
3. Treatment of health problems (stomach aches, earaches, headaches, cuts, sores, colds, coughs, ringworm, etc.)
4. Immunizations - additional consent forms are signed for <u>each</u> immunization.
5. Skin tests, blood and urine tests to detect anemia, tuberculosis, pregnancy, diabetes, high blood pressure, sexually transmitted diseases, cancer, sickle cell and other diseases.
6. Confidential treatment of sexually transmitted diseases.
7. Services related to family life responsibilities such as counseling regarding adolescent growth and development, personal responsibilities and decision-making, and family planning and contraceptive services when requested.
8. Counseling regarding problems at school and home.
9. Release of medical information to another health care agency if needed to help treat your child.
10. Treatment of your child at the clinic if a parent cannot be present.

Please circle the number of any of the services you **do not** wish your child to receive.

Please sign this form on the line below:

Parent or Guardian: _____ Date: _____

I do not want the health team to provide any services to my child.

Parent or Guardian: _____ Date: _____

If your child needs a prescription, to which pharmacy would you like it phoned?

_____   _____
Pharmacy   Phone Number

FORMA PEDIATRICA DE CONSENTIMIENTO
PARA CUIDADO PRIMARIO

Nombre del Paciente: _____ Sexo: M _____ F _____

Número de Medicaid: _____

Fecha de Nacimiento del Paciente: _____ Padres/Guardián: _____

Domicilio: _____ Número de Teléfono: _____

_____

Alergias del Paciente: _____ Número del Trabajo de los Padres: _____

Estimados Padres o Guardián:

La clínica XYZ proporciona servicios de cuidado de la salud para los adolescentes. Es necesario que usted firme esta forma para que su niño(a) reciba este tipo de cuidado. Los siguientes servicios de cuidado de la salud están disponibles:

1. Cuidado de Primeros Auxilios y Emergencias Menores.
2. Revisiones de Bienestar de Rutina y Exámenes Físicos Anuales.
3. Tratamiento de problemas de la salud (dolores de estómago, de oído, de cabeza, cortaduras, lastimaduras, resfriados, tos, tiña, y otras cosas parecidas).
4. Inmunizaciones - formas adicionales de consentimiento tendrán que ser firmadas para cada inmunización.
5. Pruebas en la piel, exámenes de sangre y orina para detectar cosas como anemia, tuberculosis, embarazo, diabetes, alta presión de la sangre, enfermedades transmitidas sexualmente, cáncer, drepanocito y otras enfermadades.
6. Tratamiento confidencial de las enfermedades transmitidas sexualmente.
7. Servicios relacionados con las responsibilidades de la vida familiar como consejería refiriéndose al crecimiento y desarrollo del adolescente, responsabilidades y decisiones personales y servicios de planeamiento familiar y anticonceptivos cuando son solicitados.
8. Consejería relacionada con problemas en la casa y en la escuela.
9. Transferir la información médica a otra agencia de cuidado de la salud si es necesario para ayudar a tratar a su niño(a).
10. Tratamiento de su niño(a) en la clínica si uno de los padres no está presente.

Por favor haga un círculo en el número de cualquiera de los servicios que usted **no desea** que que su niño(a) reciba.

Por favor firme ésta forma en la línea de abajo:

Padres o Guardián: _____ Fecha: _____

Yo no deseo que el equipo de salud proporcione ningún servicio a mi niño(a).

Padres o Guardián: _____ Fecha: _____

Si su niño(a) necesita una receta, a cuál farmacia quiere que llamen?

_____   _____

Farmacia   Número de Teléfono

EPILOGUE

. . . there is never a final grand statement and
that's the fix and the trick that works against us

—*Charles Bukowski*

Most authors like to end a work—nonfiction or fiction—in a way that capsulizes the spirit of that work. I am no exception, but we both must acknowledge that there is no single book you can open, no expert you can consult, to tell you how to be the best school nurse in your setting. Still, I believe certain general principles are universally applicable. It's up to you to translate them into specific action.

- Focus your efforts on the customer—students and parents.
- Respect diversity.
- Listen and help—don't judge. If you can't, step aside and let someone who can.
- Prevention is always the goal.
- Practice being the one-minute psychologist by paying attention to youngsters *before* problems develop; most of the "school supplies" a child needs are internal.
- Be efficient; Do the most important things first; plan ahead, stay organized, and delegate where applicable.
- Computer skills will be needed for all jobs of the future. Get ready now—take a course!
- Stay current professionally by reading nursing journals, attending seminars, and sharing experiences with peers; develop an organizational system to retrieve saved articles and notes.
- Do clinical research.
- Stay out of trouble: Know the law and nurse practice standards and document your actions.

- When dealing with tough student problems, remember the body and mind are connected; learn all you can about mental health.
- Be alert to the environment (for both hazards and benefits).
- Develop your people skills and your communication skills.
- Know your school district's mission and philosophy; familiarize yourself with the basic curriculum components. (It will empower you and give you credibility).
- Think and question.
- Don't follow trends—SET THEM!

You'll notice that many of the items on this list fall in the general area of mental health, mental abilities, or psychology. Schools and school nurses *must* pay more attention to these areas. After teaching students facts and how to think, we must find ways to help them get in touch with themselves in an honest, self-examining way: Who am I and where do I want to go? While parents and religious figures have the primary responsibility for developing spirituality in children, school personnel have a role; spirituality can and often does exist beyond religion. Remember: To students and parents, life is larger than school; development of a spiritual self helps to put the facts into perspective.